Sheri Dixon

CancerDance–
a Love story
by Sheri Dixon

ISBN-13 # 978-0-615-65898-8

I dedicate this book to my husband, Ward.
My strength, my center, my knight in shining armor.

And to my son, Alec.
Funny, smart and so very brave.
When I grow up, I wanna be just like you.

Special thanks to Alexa
For bringing order to my scattered brain.

…And we set the stage before the performance begins. The characters are introduced, not formally, but glimpsed from behind the curtain. A snippet here, a detail there; they take shape before our eyes…

1995

"How about Molly?" I asked innocently.

Months of attempting to find "the right one" for my best friend and co-worker were about to come to a startling conclusion.

Ward rolled his eyes and sighed deeply. I'd dangled every single single client in front of him since his divorce, but he'd shown no interest in any of them.

In the throes of MY divorce, I understood his reluctance to make the relationship leap again, but he was so sweet and kind- he'd made sure I was eating and taking care of myself and spent hours driving me around the countryside just to get me out to go somewhere. Most of the time I was curled up in the passenger seat…crying, so I know it wasn't for my witty personality and sparkling conversation.

Molly was substantially younger than Ward and I, but a newly minted Veterinarian and (I thought) a good intellectual and temperamental match- I knew she was honestly cheerful and good-hearted, and those were traits that would go a long way to healing my friend.

She was also drop-dead gorgeous by any standards.

"Seriously- I think she likes you, and you can't deny that she's really cute".

Ward thought about it for a minute. "Of course she's cute," he said, and unaccountably my heart flipped a little.

Without pausing, he looked straight into my eyes—not friend to friend, but man to woman—and said, "All babies are cute".

My heart flopped, and I was in love.

I had a history of choosing men that was abysmal—so much so that my employers and co-workers had informed me that before embarking on any male/female interactions I was to get their permission and blessing. And they weren't kidding.

I requested a meeting with my boss.

I said, "I've met someone I'd like to pursue a relationship with".

He said, "OK. Anyone we know?"

"Ward."

"Ward? OUR Ward?" (That Ward was also this boss' brother made it even weirder than asking my employer's permission to date already was).

"How many other Wards do we know? So—is he an acceptable candidate or not?"

I took his stunned silence as approval and beat a hasty retreat.

My first wedding back in 1979 was a huge affair- church, bridesmaids, and sit-down dinner reception- the whole nine yards. The marriage ended in 1993.

My second wedding in 1993 (see above re: terrible life choices) was at home, but with a catered meal, bakery cake and plenty of friends and family. It ended in 1995.

Ward's first marriage was a lovely yet casual affair at his parents' lakefront home in 1981 and ended in 1994.

I'm telling you all this because it's important to realize that neither one of us wanted another relationship.

I came out of my marriages tattered and shattered by abuse—I'd developed crushing anxiety attacks from the stress and the fear. I vowed I would never trust another man.

Ward came out of his marriage stunned by betrayal and abandonment- he verged on clinical depression and actually did suffer a massive heart attack requiring open-heart surgery. He vowed he would never trust another woman.

We recognized each other's pain because we lived it, slept it, saw it reflected in the other one's eyes. Being each other's best friend meant we each did everything in our power to heal, to protect, to nurture and soothe. What may have looked suspiciously like "rebound" from the outside turned out to be anything but.

His calm, gentle voice and spirit coaxed me out of the tunnel of fear, and my bullheaded determination refused to let him slip away—after his quadruple bypass I arrived at the intensive care unit and the nurse curtly asked if I was family when I said, "I need to see Ward Dixon." I waited till her eyes met mine and repeated myself quietly yet firmly, "I NEED to see Ward Dixon."

Ward's eyes opened just a bit at the touch of my hand in his. "How did you get in here?" followed by quiet laughter. "Never mind. How could they keep you out?"

We saved each other's lives, pure and simple.

1996-1998

We broke up twice.

It didn't last.

As Ward said, "I needed someone to talk to about how bad I felt, how much I hurt. I needed a best friend to talk to…but my best friend is you."

1999

On the way to work the morning of June 10th, 4 years to the day after our first official date, I stopped and picked up 2 dozen lavender Tyler roses from the lady selling them out of the back of her van.

On my break I carefully turned them into a boutonnière for Ward, a hairpiece and a bouquet for myself, and a collar corsage for the flower dog, Spooj.

At 11:30 I changed into the pretty peasant style dress I'd found at Goodwill and made sure I had the ring- my grandmother's ring- in my purse.

We met at the justice of the peace's office at noon—Ward, me, Spooj, Ward's mom and brothers. Spooj took an immediate dislike to the judge in his flowing black robe and growled through the entire 15-minute ceremony.

Then we went out for lunch at our favorite Mexican restaurant and all headed back to work.

It was my best wedding ever.

2000

"You are not allowed to let go of my hand".

After a false alarm 3 days before, I was now officially in labor.

"OK. I'll be right here".

Twelve hours later I panicked and started to cry. "I can't do it. I can't. I'm so tired. We'll have to go to the hospital".

The midwife studied Ward's face for any sign of alarm, but he remained calm. "Honey- you can do this. I know you can. But if you want to go, we will. Just say the word".

I took a nap, just a short one that muffled the pain and contractions with a blanket of exhaustion for just a few minutes.

Just under two hours after that, Alec was born at home—8 pounds 4 ounces, my 3rd child and Ward's first. I was 41 and Ward was 48.

We had planned for Ward to "catch" the baby but the midwife did it.

Because he was still holding my hand.

2001

Life took on this strange Norman Rockwell glow about it—
something I hadn't had for a very long time. Actually, being a
middle-aged newlywed and new mother was the happiest I'd ever
been.

I enjoyed my job working for my brother-in-law as the office
manager of his veterinary clinic, and later became the manager for
the emergency clinic that was owned by 19 area veterinarians.

Ward was working for an auto parts importer as inventory
manager.

Alec was a joy and a wonder.

Our old house (circa 1890) was getting renovated—one room, one
project at a time.

I was slowly rebuilding the little 3 acre farm I'd had in Wisconsin
on our little 3 acre farm in East Texas—Arabian horse, dairy goats,
dogs, cats, a room full of pedigreed long-haired guinea pigs, and
we'd added some poultry for good measure.

Our home was filled with love, and laughter, and security, and
normalcy.

Of course it couldn't last.

**...In the background the music begins, so quietly the dancers
aren't even aware of it yet.**

Most of the rest of this story is told in journal form, directly transferred from a thread on an online forum. In the beginning, the intent of the entries were merely transfer of information, but it quickly shifted into a therapeutic exercise—the internet being just anonymous enough to let me vent my anger and frustrations, but just personal enough to really feel like we were surrounded by friends.

And we ARE surrounded by friends. What doesn't show here are the hundreds—no, thousands—of replies and comments made by people literally around the world—people who prayed for us in every language and to every imaginable god, who sent us good wishes, energies, and tangible gifts.

In 2010 I started a blog, so some of those entries are in here as well, tucked in chronologically.

Before the journal entries, there is one final introductory bit - the incidents that started this whole thing a decade ago, but that I didn't bother to record at the time, because at the time those events were supposed to be short-lived and boring, and where's the value in remembering THAT?

The title, "CancerDance," is because we're not alone in this—in fact, we're experiencing a very mild exposure.

Just being in the whole doctor/testing/hospital/lab maze has been horrifying and humbling, and the faces who surround us there are carbon copies of our own fear, impotence, and resignation at following the same steps over and over again, all of us moving and bending to the routines and the schedules, the stresses and the worries.

Praying that even though we hate the melody, that the dance will end on a good note…

…If only we can dance long enough.

The curtain opens- the dancers are in place and the lights come up.

Cue the music.

2002

All good stories start out one of two ways, so I'll combine them and start this one:

Once upon a time, it was a dark and stormy night...

"What's that thing on your eyelid?" I asked my husband. "Nothing—just a little stye," he answered and went back to his book.

The Nothing stayed virtually unchanged over the next year or so, but then Ward started having trouble with his eye. The stye looked the same, but the lid seemed to be pushing out just enough to disallow full closure of the eye, causing dryness and scratchiness.

The eye doctor seemed unconcerned and did a biopsy, which came back and was reported casually. "Just a little skin cancer—we can cut that out in office with Mohs Microsurgery and with minimum or no disfigurement."

On the day of the procedure (we didn't even think of it as surgery), we arrived at the clinic and were told that they'd be taking thin slices of the affected area, freezing them, and then looking under the microscope while we waited. If the margins weren't clear— free of cancer cells—they'd call him back and do it again till they were. Easy.

First go around, we weren't surprised when they called him back— since it was on his eyelid and there's not a lot of baggy skin there to play with, they were taking very tiny slices to avoid the need for any major reconstructive surgery.

Eight hours later, they'd called him back multiple times—I stopped counting at 6—and by the time they sent him home heavily sedated, Ward had an opening that started where the stye had been and continued halfway around to his ear. Under the dressing, that entire side of the eyeball was clearly visible apparently held in place only by the optic nerve.

The 'little skin cancer' had had tentacles, and what we'd seen on the surface was literally the tip of the iceberg.

"No matter", they told us. "We got it all. Not even a need for radiation. Go to the cataract clinic for your reconstruction tomorrow and have a nice life."

The next day the surgeon looked at Ward and said, "My, you had a hard time yesterday. Today will be easy. I'll just put you to sleep and you'll wake up in 45 minutes all done."

I was confident enough in her words that I took her advice and went to get myself some lunch while they were in surgery.

Forty-five minutes later I returned to the clinic and sat down in the waiting room. I cocked my head with a trace of concern when I heard sirens, then realized how paranoid I was being—we WERE across the street from two regional hospitals…

Just then the nurse came out. "Mrs. Dixon?" she asked.

I got up, smiled and said, "All done, huh?"

The nurse looked at me hard and said quietly, "You need to come with me."

The door closed behind me, but all I could see was the room in front of me—my Ward, on the stretcher, surrounded by the doctor, the nurses, the firemen, and EMT's. They were all hollering at him to stay still, to calm down while they tried to place a breathing tube in him, and he was fighting them like a Big Dog. The nurse next to me seemed to be whispering, but I'm pretty sure she was almost yelling to be heard over everything else.

"I'm sorry, Mrs. Dixon. When the doctor got him fully under anesthetic, his heart stopped".

You read it in books and see it in movies, but I'd never actually seen anyone fall to the ground in surprise and grief, much less done it myself. But it happens.

When your world falls out from under you, it happens.

~ ~ ~

Three days. Ward had been in the hospital for three days and not seen a doctor yet.

I was ferrying between my job, caring for the house and our two-year-old son (who was staying with neighbors during all this), and spending every other minute—waking or sleeping—in the hospital. Every day I asked when the doctor would be in and every day I was told that they had him on a heart monitor and the PAs (Physician's Assistants) were coming in to see him—everything was under control.

I was there when the last PA came in.

He marched into the room, all full of himself and professional, pretending to read Ward's chart. He never once looked at Ward.

"Mr. Dixon, I see you came in through the emergency room. Were you having chest pains?"

I spoke as quietly and calmly as I could manage.

"No. He was not having chest pains. If you'll truly READ the chart, you'll see that Mr. Dixon was in the process of being anesthetized for surgery at the cataract center when his HEART STOPPED, and if you'll truly LOOK at Mr. Dixon, you'll see that he's got a HUGE HONKIN' HOLE IN HIS HEAD WHERE THEY STILL NEED TO DO THE SURGERY ONCE WE CAN GET A REAL **DOCTOR** IN HERE TO TELL THEM HOW TO PROCEED."

Not waiting for a reply, I strode to the nurses' station and told them "My husband has been here THREE days, without his meds, and with an open surgical site. He needs to see a cardiologist NOW. It's right around lunchtime. If you can't find one for him, I will go down to the cafeteria, which is CRAWLING with doctors, and drag one up here myself."

Thirty minutes later, the cardiologist came into the room—still in surgical scrubs. He LOOKED at both of us, shook our hands, and sat on the side of the bed.

"I'm so very sorry, Mr. and Mrs. Dixon—until 30 minutes ago, I didn't even know you were here".

In an hour, they'd done an EKG.

At 10pm that night, after an already full day of surgeries, he was placing the two stents needed to open Ward's arteries—they were almost 100% closed, and Ward had had no symptoms.

If Ward's heart had stressed anywhere else—the day surgery clinic during that grueling eight hours, at work, driving our son to the babysitter's, anywhere that there weren't cardiac paddles literally in reach, he would've died.

Within a week, we were back in surgery— at the main hospital and with a cardiac anesthesiologist in attendance—and the hole in Ward's head was finally closed up.

Our new best friend, the cardiologist, set up a schedule to aggressively and pro-actively monitor Ward's heart—he'd had that quadruple bypass years before and his family practice doctor had been kind of lackadaisical about watching for heart problems.

We knew better now, and it would not happen again.

The surgery site healed without incident, and we took the doctor's words to heart—we went home to have a nice life.

And for four years, it was.

2006

May 2 2006, 09:31 AM

My husband of 7 years (it took me three tries to get a good one) is facing aggressive cancer surgery next week. This is a recurrence of a cancer they removed (or MOSTLY removed, it turns out) four years ago.

Then it was on his eyelid and some of the muscle around the eye.

Now it's everywhere in that area and they are going to remove the entire muscle, the eyeball, the lids, all the tissue surrounding it, and some bone as well. There will be three surgeons working on it, and they are taking a skin graft from his leg to cover the big gaping hole they will make removing a quarter of his face.

They don't 'think' it's traveled to the brain or jaw, but they won't be sure till they get in there.

This is not a cancer that responds to chemo or radiation.

The whole thing stinks, and I'm angry as hell.

My husband is a quiet gentle soul and would never complain or shake his fist at the heavens.

That's MY job

We have a six-year-old boy.

We were looking at bigger pieces of land to move our house to.

We were finally getting our heads above water financially after his last two hospitalizations (he has diabetes and heart issues also).

Ya, I KNOW everything happens for a reason, but where's the sense in THIS?

General consensus is that being married to me should be punishment enough for any wrongs he committed in this life or ANY previous ones.

Poop.

May 5 2006, 09:26 PM

We went for the stress test today. They did the EKG and sent Ward directly to the doctor—no stress test.

It seems that he has a big ol' hairy clot at the top of his heart that needs to be blasted with blood thinners ASAP. Unfortunately, he also has that pesky cancer that needs to be cut off ASAP.

-If they thin his blood, they can't cut on the cancer
-If they take the cancer, the anesthetic may stress his heart and he could throw the clot. (Bad, they tell me.)

They 'think' he'll be stable enough for surgery, so the plan is to proceed with the cancer surgery on Thursday with the assistance of a cardiac anesthesiologist instead of a regular one.

Then, once the giant hole where his eye used to be is healed sufficiently, they will blast him with Coumadin and hope that it dissolves the clot.

In the midst of this one of my best friends called to say that her 20-year-old son's body was found. He'd been shot in the back of the head, execution style. I've known this boy since he was ten and he's the same age as my older boy.

(For some reason, I seem to be covered in stress-induced hives...itchy itchy itchy...)

May 10 2006, 12:54 PM

Surgery is tomorrow at 1pm CST.

Last night we were out feeding the animals and Ward manually lifted his eyelid, looked out into the forest, and said, "Take a last look, little guy".

Our six-year-old son insists on going with us to the hospital, and I can't bear to banish him for the day—his dad is his whole life.

This is breaking my heart.

May 11 2006, 9:45PM

I'm home and very tired.

The surgery went well—only an hour-and-a-half instead of the three or four hours they thought it would be.

The cancer was well defined and easy to take out and the pathology lab said all the margins were clear.

Ward's heart remained well behaved through the whole thing (which was the main thing I was worried about—that pesky cancer thing was incidental).

They took about a 6-by-6 inch graft from his leg for the repair and said that would probably be the ouchiest part of healing.

When we left him he was in his room, chocolate pudding in one hand and his morphine-on-demand button in the other.

For the moment, life is good.

I came home, fed the critters and the boy, and once I email and/or call all of our friends and family, I'm off to bed.

Maybe some cocoa first...

May 19 2006, 11:08 AM

We went for the first post-op appointment yesterday and they took the packing out of his face.

They said his leg looks about how they usually do (yicky), but that the face graft IS taking (healing). We were REALLY worried about that since he's a diabetic.

We need to keep it lubed up and covered with a loose gauze pad and go back on Monday.

They took him off of antibiotics and Vicadin (he's so sad about that...)

May 20 2006, 09:31 PM

His leg is very ouchy still and looks pretty rough, but where his eye used to be doesn't hurt hardly at all and for that we are thankful—he spent the better part of the last six months in pain from it.

Tomorrow I get to help change the dressing, and we'll see how bad it is. He said the little bit he saw in the doctor's office was creepy looking—he said it's just a really deep socket covered with skin...

May 21 2006, 01:45 PM

It was way worse than I was prepared for.

It's almost twice as big as I thought and twice as deep and very black—I'm hoping because it's healing and not because the graft is dying.

It's literally just a big black socket—the kind you'd see in a horror movie except this is REAL and attached to my beloved husband.

The doctor should be able to tell us more tomorrow.

He told me not to help, but I told him I at least wanted to see it. Then I had to leave the room and have felt just sick ever since.

My poor baby.

At least he said it doesn't hurt at all.

17 years in animal emergency medicine seeing everything and this was the worst.

Bleah.

Jun 10 2006, 11:11 PM

An update:

Ward's leg is healed up nicely, but his surgery site is infected so he's back on antibiotics.

The doctor said that he needs to leave the patch off as much as possible, since that's what set him up for infection—the warm moist environment under the patch.

He just won't do it—he's so afraid Alec will see him and be permanently repulsed by his looks.

He finally let me look at it again and it's not as shocking as the first peek, although it is clearly infected.

He NEEDS to let air get at it, or he'll be back in the hospital with the infection.

Strength and patience.

I need strength and patience.

Jun 11 2006, 12:55 AM

Poor Ward is having a hard time reconciling the new face he sees in the mirror with the face he used to have.

Alec had a bad revelation yesterday—apparently he thought the eye would grow back.

It's just a difficult time all around, made worse by this infection.

Jun 19 2006, 10:06 AM

AARRRGGGHHHH!!!!

We are scheduled to go on vacation in August. It's been planned for a year. The work and travel schedules of my grown children, my parents, some dear friends and myself have been altered to accommodate it. I haven't seen my 75-year-old dad in 2 years and my dear friends in almost 7. One set of friends we are supposed to visit has scheduled their WEDDING for when we can be there. We have reservations at a small family-owned resort on a lake for which we have paid a non-refundable deposit. I have made arrangements for all the animals here to be cared for.

Last week Ward's boss said, "You know, you've taken so much time off for this cancer thing, and now we are getting a new computer system which you will be integral in instituting the last week of July—so YOU CAN'T GO."

I called this boss person (I was nice even though it almost kilt me) and explained that BECAUSE of what Ward's been through he really needs the vacation and that he'd come in early/stay late before and after to get the computer stuff done. I also reminded him that Ward's been there 7 years and never ever taken advantage of time off. If he's not there, he's in the hospital.
I told him we really need the 5 days off that he is due (he took all his hospital time without pay). He said the most he could spare him would be 3 days.

Now that SEEMS like a small difference but 5 days would have a weekend on each side, so 9 days altogether. 3 days is only one weekend, so 5 days altogether.

If we drive like bats outta you know where, we could make the cabin part and see my older kids. We could spend one evening with my folks. Everything else would have to be eliminated.

Ward's boss said, "Why don't you fly Ward up to the cabin part and back, and you and Alec drive the rest?" Well, first of all, that's an extra $300 we just don't have, and second of all that would mean 4,000 miles alone in the car WITH A SIX YEAR OLD. Is he INSANE???

I go from being resigned to just the 5 days, to pushing this guy a little more (I can't believe he'd be dumb enough to fire Ward over 16 hours of work. He knows Ward is planning on staying there till retirement 11 years from now and anyone he hires new will have to be trained and people just don't have company loyalty like they used to), to looking for a new job altogether for Ward.

I know this seems trivial and silly, but dang it—my husband AND his family NEED some time off that we aren't spending at the hospital.

Jul 5 2006, 09:58 AM

Well it's still all up in the air.

I have pigheadedly made hotel reservations with the knowledge that I can cancel if I need to, but trying to find them last minute would've been hard.

After exhausting all ideas, we found out that if he quits or gets fired his employer must insure him for six months with him paying the full premium. Then he can go on my insurance, which will have to take his pre-existings since he will have had no break in coverage.

Of course it will be very expensive for both options.

We are trying to be sensible about this and are looking for a different job for Ward (with insurance) so he can give notice at this place, go on vacation, and start a new one when he gets back.

If that doesn't work, we'll go to plan B.

(Now I've gotta THINK of a plan B....)

The doctor said his surgery site (can't say 'eye', and can't bring myself to say 'socket') is healing well. She wants to see him in another 2 weeks and will set him up with the oncologist for radiation.

I'm sure THAT will throw yet another monkey wrench into the whole picnic...

Jul 8 2006, 10:22 AM

Well, last night Alec was in the shower and he called his dad in there for something (to identify a spider in the bathroom—when you have an old house the bathroom is your own little nature preserve) and Ward unthinkingly went in there without his eye covered,

Which he realized when he saw Alec's face.

Alec bravely said, "I'm fine. I didn't even feel like throwing up".

I wish Ward were as optimistic.

Aug 13 2006, 02:29 PM

We went on 'vacation'—3032 miles from Friday night to Thursday lunchtime.
Ward's boss didn't budge on giving him only 3 days instead of the 5 he put in for a YEAR ago, but he did say he didn't have to be back till lunchtime Thursday.

What a peach.

We didn't get to see most of the friends we had wanted to on the way up and back, including the wedding we were supposed to attend and the 20 hours up and 20 hours back were grueling- I'd drive for 4 hours, then sleep while Ward drove for 2 hours, then he'd sleep while I drove. Alec listened to Dragon Rider on tape— narrated by Brendon Fraser and an excellent story.

Our visit with the older kids and our dear friends in Minnesota was wonderful, and our cabin was so right on the lake that we could wake up in the morning and see the lake directly outside the window and hear the loons calling. It was lovely and green and

COOL at night, so different from East Texas right now where we consider it a plus if it drops below 80 at night.
Of course, in the winter I'll be in bare feet here while our friends will be wearing snowshoes, so I'll still take East Texas.

Ward is sleeping most all the time, which is a worry, and tomorrow he starts 6 weeks (30 treatments) of radiation, which will wear him down even more.

Because of his boss, he's going to try to work through the radiation, but I know he won't make it.

I told Ward that the man would work him till he had to roll his body out of the way for the next guy to take his desk, and he agrees, but we NEED the insurance and everything we've done to do 'right' has just worked against us:

-He went right back to work after having his EYE removed; therefore he probably won't qualify for disability.

-I fought long and hard for health insurance where *I* work, and now he won't qualify for the TX high risk pool because he 'could' get insurance through me—even though it will be way more expensive than the high risk pool.

-Even though we've been paying the 'credit life and disability' insurance on our debts for just this occasion, since he's back at WORK, it won't kick in even though he's missing so much through treatments and appointments and having to pay the co-pays for all those while losing pay from work.

Tomorrow is another day, and I need to start back the fight to figure out just how we are going to financially, mentally and physically survive this.

On August 19, 2006, we looked at a piece of property—roughly the 13,426th piece we'd looked at in the 4 years after our "Pesky little cancer is gone; have a nice life" directive from the local doctor back in 2002.

Looking at land may have seemed frivolous considering everything else, but it was something that we could do that was concrete, forward-looking, and positive—I absolutely refused to consider that our plans as a family for our future would be eradicated by disease.

Our dreams may need to be adjusted for reality, and delayed some, but never, ever, EVER given up on.

The difficult part was staying within our specific parameters of location, topography, size and price.

This piece turned out to be IT—and being able to "Go Home" became a driving force for all of us.

2007

May 30 2007, 12:16 PM

So today Ward went for his 'yearly follow-up' visit to the plastic surgeon who put his face back together and the surgeon did a BIOPSY on a 'suspicious area'.

Not a 'routine just making sure there's no cancer hiding' biopsy.

A 'this area is not healing like the rest of it and looks problematic' biopsy.

IF the cancer is back, they've already taken his eye and all the surrounding muscle and tissue and bone.

The only places for it to go now are his nasal cavity, his jaw, or his brain.

...I'm not feeling so well right now...

Jun 3 2007, 09:22 PM

His doctor called late Friday afternoon to tell us that the results were NOT back yet and I give him 100 points for doing that himself and not having a nurse do it or just blowing it off.

We had to be out of town for the weekend, which was a good diversion.

Hopefully (?) tomorrow...

04 June 2007 at 10:45pm

We found out about five hours ago that Ward's cancer is back—same cancer, same place.

Since it's now evaded:
-The Mohs Microsurgery (so detailed that they didn't even bother with radiation 5 years ago- checked, rechecked, triple checked and proclaimed him cured)

-Radical disfiguring surgery to remove the cancer and ALL surrounding tissue, muscle and bone, checking to make sure they had clean margins and THEN

-Just to be extra sure frying it with 6 weeks of radiation and again proclaiming him cured one year ago,

They've referred him to MDAnderson Cancer Center in Houston, and are fast-tracking all his records there.

Apparently, this kind of cancer does not normally spread to other areas of the body, but can be 'problematic and aggressive locally'.

Ya THINK?

We pretty much feel like the whole planet's been pulled out from under us.

08 June 2007 at 10:53pm

Today:

-We got the records from the cardiologist faxed to MDA.

-We got the records from the radiation oncologist faxed to MDA.

-We gave the scheduler enough verbal history so that she could go on and email the doctor for a definite appointment—should hear back on that by Monday sometime.

-We found a hotel that accepts pets (our terrier, Spooj) and is well under $100 per night.

-We found a doggie daycare that's right up the street from MDA and will be cheaper than boarding her HERE, and she'll be able to come to the hotel with us at night.

-We found out that there is a Kids' Room for Alec to go to when he can't be with us (he said "I'll go, but if anyone asks if I'm not too old to be in daycare, I'm telling them that I'm being held against my will").

-My employees have offered to take care of Alec's kitty there at the clinic for us so we don't have to pay to board her either.

-I was worried about asking my neighbor to take care of all the other critters for that long—she's just started working full time—but her granddaughter (teenager) will be coming to spend the summer a few days before we leave and LOVES the animals. So we'll be training her to do it under Patsy's supervision, and my other adult neighbor, Patsy's sister-in-law, will supervise on the days Patsy needs to leave extra early.

-I've arranged for our bookkeeper at work to take care of payroll if we have to be gone over a payday and will get her all the 'just in case' stuff before we leave.

-My full-time doctor has offered to do all the drug orders (He said, "No problem—there's a cute $500 retractor I've had my eye on...").

-Ward's boss is still ok with the whole thing and (amazingly) there was a raise in his paycheck today **and** he's been told they are hiring an assistant for him (I told him to insist on a cute young one with big...intellects) in case he needs to be off for an extended period. (Granted, he's needed both raise and help for over a year now—every time someone else quits they load all THEIR stuff on Ward).

10 June 2007 at 8:39am

Today is our 8th anniversary.

My first two weddings were big fancy affairs, but in retrospect, I should have taken more care in choosing the grooms than planning the ceremonies.

This wedding was about as casual as you can get, but the groom's a keeper.

12 June 2007 at 11:19pm

Well, we have an official approved appointment at MDA for next Tuesday with the doctor whose area of interest is orbital tumors.

Ward had his 'routine' (gads that word gives me the willies) stress test and echocardiogram and the clot that was on his heart a year ago has reformed—not as in "is now behaving," but as in it's there again—so he's back on Coumadin and they'll have to be REALLY careful if they decide to take a 'let's cut him open' attitude.

...It's always something...

So we'll drive down on Monday, get checked into our hotel, and do a practice drive from the hotel to the daycare to the hospital.

I mapquested it and it's supposedly 3 hours 44 minutes from our front door to the hotel (Homestead Studio Suites—a one room efficiency with kitchenette. They accept pets and have a special MDA rate), 6 minutes from the hotel to the daycare (Doggy daycare for Spooj. Ironically, I think her digs will be snazzier than ours.), and 9 minutes from the doggy daycare to the hospital.

I talked to the insurance company again today and got a 'worst case scenario' of out-of-pocket expenses and although it's bad, it's not insurmountable.

Adding that to the travel/staying expenses is brushing up against insurmountable, especially if they decide to do surgery and our stay pushes at or over two weeks instead of one, but I think it'll be all right.

It'll have to be.

13 June 2007 at 10:54pm

%$^&*&$$%^&^%%$^$#!!!!!!!

Sorry.

Just a whole day of conflicting information and stupid roadblocks.

14 June 2007 at 9:01pm

Today—better.

We have what I hope are final answers and good direction.

As of TODAY:

The insurance has been verified and all we'll owe at time of service is our co-pays. The business office supervisor who I talked to has put in the file to bill the rest out after we're all done (not thinking that far ahead *shudder*).

We are going down yonder on Monday afternoon so we can avoid rush hour traffic but still do a 'dry run' to find where all we need to go the next morning.
Tuesday we are to be at the hospital at 6am to register Ward, then they take him back for his MRI. At that point, Alec and I will take Spooj (patiently waiting in the car in the parking garage—should still be cool enough at that time of day) to the doggie daycare, which opens at 7am. We'll come back to the hospital and Alec will go to the kids' room that opens at 8am and I'll go find Ward to accompany him to his first doctor's appointment at 9:30am.

Anything beyond that is an unknown.

Wheeeeee...

14 June 2007 at 11:12pm

I just printed out the forms we need to fill out to take with us-

Eight pages for Ward to fill out for MD Anderson, world-renowned cancer center.

Five pages for Spooj to fill out for Midtown Doggy Daycare.

Seriously.

17 June 2007 at 11:54pm

Spent today making lists, gathering stuff, checking the lists off, then remembering OTHER lists I've gotta make and gather stuff for...

In addition to the stuff we'll need to take for our dubious vacation of undisclosed time frame, we have:

-Alec's tournament in Beaumont next Saturday, for which I had to sew his new personalized patch on the back of his uniform top (tres tough).

-There's a woman coming up from Victoria to pick up 3 little guinea pigs (their sale will finance us for a day) so THEY had to be bathed and their pedigrees typed up. A Houston-based guinea pig friend is coming to the hotel to pick them up and will hold them for 'Victoria Lady' so we don't have to mess with anything but getting them from here to the hotel.

-Of course Spooj needed to be as UNcountrified as possible—she's deflea-ed, un-matted, and smells like L'oreal Vanilla Crème shampoo. She's brilliant white and all poofy—ready to hobnob with the Downtown Houston Yuppie Puppies.

I've also mapquested every possible trip, route, and side trip we may take or WANT to take while there, along with printing off info on the Houston Zoo, Museum of Natural Science, and Aquarium.

All the numbers I may need are in my little black book.

We did take Ward out for Chinese tonight for Father's Day...

Tomorrow we'll be up and out by the crack of nine to deliver the house pets who won't be traveling with us- Tiny Ramon the geriatric poodle and Alec's cat, Saphira- the Kitten From Hell to their appointed caregivers, make one last stop at work, take some guinea pigs to the pet store, drop off bookkeeping, run to the post office, and, in our SPARE TIME before lunch, wash the car and get the yearly inspection done.

Then home for lunch, packing the stuff we've stacked in the family room, loading the car, and heading out when Ward gets home around 2ish.

On the way to the hospital for our appointments I had a meltdown. Full-blown, absolute panic attack.

I don't know if it was cumulative stress, or the fact that I was worried we'd be late, or that we'd done the 'dry run' the night before but that only took us TO the hospital—once inside we had no idea how to navigate the miles of buildings, floors and corridors—or maybe just because I'm a little mentally unstable by nature, but halfway there (and it's a very short trip) I announced to Ward, "Stop the car. I've gotta get out."

Ward: What? Honey, we're almost there.
Me: STOP THE CAR. I'VE GOTTA GET OUT NOW.
Ward: Honey? I can see the hospital just ahead...
Me: Lemme out lemme out lemme out lemme out...

Alec: Mom? Are you going to throw up? Do you need the trashcan?
Ward:- It's OK, A-man. Your mom's just having a little break down. She'll be fine as soon as she can get out of the car in the parking garage.

And I was.

19 June 2007 at 7:26pm

Today:

Getting around is MUCH easier than I anticipated—once downtown, we don't have to do anything but city streets and, even when busy, I don't find those as scary as the freeways.
Alec had a blast in the Kids' Room—didn't even notice for a full five minutes when we came to get him after FOUR hours (he and a new friend the same age were video-gaming). Spooj's Executive Condo is as nice as our hotel room (and our room is very nice—not fancy, but clean and serviceable). MDAnderson itself is HUGE, with patients from all over the world, which is comforting.

Now.

Ward so far has two doctors working on his case—both commented on the weight of his file... They seem very competent and have a special interest in this type and placement of cancer.

Our worst little surprise of the morning was that in reviewing the chart, the doctor said, "So when they did the enucleation, the margins were still positive…"

And I said, "NO. They kept him under anesthesia while they sent the tumor to the lab so they wouldn't close without clear margins."

He said, "Well, on the surgery date, they WERE determined clear BUT the final pathology report came back later as POSITVE."

POSITIVE

POSITIVE

In June. And they didn't irradiate till SEPTEMBER.

We are physically sick about this. Completely.

The doctors couldn't believe they didn't tell us.

And we've always been told it's just 'basal cell', but what the biopsy shows is that it's a rare, locally very aggressive subtype called Morpheaform. Even sounds nasty. These cells are very narrow and tiny and are usually UNDER estimated as far as spread. (Ya THINK???)

So the plan now is:

-He had an MRI, EKG, blood work and chest x-ray (cuz of the clot in his heart) this morning.

-They are scheduling a CAT scan to see if it's in the bone or just the tissue.

-Then he needs to see the Cardiologist down here since the surgery will probably be at least 8 hours long and they don't want to 'compromise' his heart while killing the cancer.

-Surgery is the only way to go, since they said he already almost maxed out on 'safe' radiation a year ago. (?)

-Then a plastic surgeon consult because of his diabetes and healing issues with a new and 'extensive' area to re-build.

-Then a consult with a researcher to see if he'd qualify for a clinical trial of some new drug—not usually used for this type of cancer, but the doctors thought it may help.

Then surgery.

Then a long, long recovery.

I really just wanna go home now...

20 June 2007 at 10:38pm

Today:

No doctors—they've (so far) set us up with the appointment with the doctor who specializes in pre-surgical risk cases and his CAT scan for tomorrow. Today we went to the Downtown Aquarium, which was very cool and took our minds off of 'stuff' for a while.

Spooj went back to doggy daycare while we aquarium-ed and it's the first place I've ever left her that she comes out looking happy. I picked up a flyer from the front desk and here's one of the (honest to goodness) options for boarding dogs:

"The Paw-perfect Doggy Package" includes two extra playtimes, ten minutes of pool time, a suite treat, a bedtime story, an ice cream break, and bottled instead of tap water."

Only an extra $25 per day...

Needless to say, Spooj is NOT signed up for that, but her new friend Farouq admits that her wiry, expressive eyebrows waggling at him forlornly have earned her an ice cream break in the afternoons.

21 June 2007 at 8:51pm

Today we went to the Museum of Natural Science and then the appointment with the internist who is adjusting Ward's medications to make him all strong and whatnot for surgery. He spent over an hour with us, reviewing the records, doing an exam, and taking history. Very detailed.

Tonight (at *9pm*) he has his CAT scan and then we are DONE at MDA for the time being.

We need to be back here on Friday July 6th for appointments with:
-The research doctor
-The cardiologist
-The anesthesiologist
-The plastic surgeon (appointment pending)
-The surgeons we saw on Tuesday

And he's scheduled for surgery on Monday July 9th. I expect we'll be here that whole week.

Since we have Alec's tournament in Beaumont on Saturday, it would be wasteful to drive home tonight and back down here tomorrow night, so I guess we will just have to suck it up and spend the day at the beach on Galveston Island tomorrow (heavy sigh/tired smile).

Since Alec doesn't compete till late afternoon Saturday, Spooj will have to spend Saturday night at doggy daycare and they aren't open for pick up till 4pm Sunday, so we'll go to the Medical Museum and ride the metro rail (Alec's request) from our hotel across from the Astrodome to downtown and back, pick up the Spoojer and head HOME Sunday evening.

Yay.

21 June 2007 at 10:52pm

Alec. (Sigh.)

I think it's because he's Ward's only child and he appeared late in life, but he and Ward are so close, and Ward's parenting style has always been to treat Alec as another person, instead of a kid. Even a year ago, Alec insisted that he go to the hospital with us on surgery day and sat in that waiting room like a trooper. He wouldn't even hear of staying behind this time. So we've made every effort to do 'normal family stuff' in between the very abnormal hospital stuff.

And he's got his dad's brain—he was explaining to us this afternoon the difference between physical, emotional and spiritual.

He's SEVEN.

Luckily (?) they both also have a really strange, well-exercised sense of humor—so while Alec is growing up perhaps faster than other kids, he's also keeping Ward years younger than if he had remained childless.

...Just another worry for ol' mom...

22 June 2007 at 9:45pm

Finally got to my beloved Galveston today. We were waylaid by phone calls and appointment problems (the plastic surgeon our surgeon wants is ONLY available to see us on THIS Wednesday-so we'll be driving home Sunday, and then making a quick trip back TWO DAYS LATER—ten total hours of driving for 15 minutes with the plastic surgeon, but if THAT'S the guy who will make Ward's recovery work, then THAT'S the guy we're going to.

The internist's consultations with Ward's primary doctor back home made him decide to give him a special med to bring his potassium levels down—they are apparently rising quick enough to cause concern for his liver—and he wanted him starting it TODAY. They called while we were on our way to Galveston and they wanted it started so quickly that they called it to a pharmacy in Galveston. So we went there and waited.

And waited.

And waited.

I could SEE the ocean. I could SMELL the ocean. I could HEAR the ocean... after FORTY minutes, the little gal behind the counter said, "I'm sorry—we have to order that- it'll be here first thing in the morning."

If anyone on this hemisphere heard an explosion—that was me.

After the smoke cleared, I called the doctor back and they asked if we could make it to the hospital pharmacy by 8pm.

Sure.

Why not?

So we went to the beach, saw crabs, Alec fed the seagulls his lunch sandwich; we played in the water, and gathered shells.

And got to the MDA pharmacy at 7:30pm—sandy, smelling like seaweed, but in time.

When we come down on the 5th, all our appointments are on the 6th and then we'll have the weekend before surgery on the 9th and we ARE BY GUM going to spend that weekend on the beach.

Gotta get that boy showered, his hair cut, and his uniform laid out cuz tomorrow is the tournament....

23 June 2007 at 9:43pm

Southeastern Regional Conference Tournament

Jr. Greenbelt Sparring Bronze Medal:

Alec Dixon, Brownsboro TX

24 June 2007 at 11:23pm

We're home

26 June 2007 at 10:11am

It IS nice being home.

Whoops.

Time to go...

We're driving back down tonight for our appointment tomorrow morning.

Be back tomorrow night late.

Then we get to stay home a whole WEEK (woo hoo).

27 June 2007 at 11:55pm

Back home...again...for a week and a day.

We met the plastic surgeon today and are feeling very good about the surgery now. The cancer surgeon is (his official Bio):

"Ehab Hanna, M.D., FACS, is an internationally recognized head and neck surgeon and expert in the treatment of patients with Skull Base Tumors and Head and Neck cancer. He is Professor and Vice Chair of the Department of Head and Neck Surgery at The University of Texas M. D. Anderson Cancer Center in Houston, Texas. After earning his medical degree, he completed a surgery internship at Vanderbilt University, and residency in Otolaryngology-Head and Neck Surgery at The Cleveland Clinic in Cleveland, Ohio. He received advanced fellowship training in skull base surgery and head and neck surgical oncology at the University of Pittsburgh Medical Center. He joined the M. D. Anderson faculty in 2004, with a joint appointment at Baylor College of Medicine. He is the medical director of the Multidisciplinary Head and Neck Center, and co-director of the Skull Base Tumor program at MD Anderson. He is also leading the development of minimally invasive and robotic applications in skull base surgery. Dr. Hanna has consistently been named one of America's Top Doctors by the Castle Connolly Guide. In addition to patient care, Dr. Hanna is actively engaged in clinical and translational research with emphasis on skull base tumors. He is the Editor-in-Chief of the journal of *Head & Neck*, which is the official journal of the International Federation of Head and Neck Societies. He also co-edited a textbook on 'Comprehensive Management of Skull Base Tumors.'"

And the plastic surgeon will be (official Bio again):

"Dr. Matthew Hanasono, M.D. performs reconstructive surgery for patients with cancer involving all areas of the body. His clinical interests include reconstructive surgery for patients with head and neck cancer, breast cancer, and cancer of the upper and lower extremities. Within head and neck cancer, Dr. Hanasono specializes in complex reconstruction of the face, oral cavity, upper and lower jaws, and skull base, including the facial nerve. Dr. Hanasono has performed hundreds of micro vascular free flap surgeries for cancer patients. He also performs reconstructions after removal of skin cancers, such as after Moh's surgery or surgery for melanoma."

I think I actually believe THESE guys when they say it's gonna be OK and it's gonna STAY OK after they are done with him.

I'm just very tired (last 24 hours—10 hours driving, 5 hours sleeping, 4 hours at the hospital, 6 hours packing, unpacking, and taking care of critters) and overwhelmed with everything that ISN'T getting done, that HAS to get done, and that I'm afraid WON'T get done—primarily getting this place clean enough to bring my post-op hubby into. I'm not even worried about 'neat' (although our cumulative packrattedness is starting to get to even me). I'm worried about Ward in a 100+ year old house that's hard for me to clean with 12' ceilings and 8' windows.

No central A/C, so that's dust coming in through the screens and our little creepy crawly friends who find their way in.

Diabetic with several large wounds + the above house = bad.

29 June 2007 at 7:00pm

Hey—I normally am not worried about my lack of housekeeping skills. It's just the germ-thing with Ward and all—he's gonna have the main surgery site on his head that'll be, ummmmm, big.

They are taking tissue from his forearm to fill the head hole.

Then they are taking skin from his thigh to cover the arm hole.

They will be taking a CHUNK of tissue to fill in the socket this time instead of the simple skin flap they did last time that left just a big, well.... socket that was a good atmosphere for pockets of ick to sit in.

For reasons unknown to me, being a simple non-medical gal, the forearm has better "eye socket tissue" than the thigh.

Also unlike the skin flap, they will be pulling in one of the chewing muscles (they said we have 10, so he'll be ok and not like...droop or drool) and then microscopically connect blood vessels and whatnot. He'll have an incision going partly down his neck to pull those up and in.

Pretty

03 July 2007 at 1:27am

Today's been...busy. Things I thought were in order at work have turned out to be so NOT, which is really cutting into the time I needed to take to make this house clean enough for Ward to recover in.

I'm just NOW (at midnight o'clock) finished with the kitchen—I started at 6:30pm after already spending three hours on it yesterday. Luckily, Ward helped with the tall stuff—those 12' ceilings are a bitch to get the cobwebs off of...
GOOD things:

-The doctors and staff I work for and with took up a secret kitty and presented me with an envelope containing $850—enough to pay all our out-of-pocket expenses next week.

-My friend, who lives just up the road from us and who I was planning on buying hay from this year, said she didn't put into the secret kitty, but that there WERE going to be 25 bales of hay tucked into my barn by the hay fairy to start us out for the season.

-Knowing that I was going to be all by myself with Alec on Monday, my bestest friend in the world, Cathy, who I've known for 27 years, called me tonight to tell me that they are going to Colorado from tomorrow through Sunday night, but Monday morning she's getting a flight from Dallas to Houston and will be at the hospital by 9am—where she will stay with us till about 9pm.

I'm tired, but really feeling my blessings today...

05 July 2007 at 1:16am

The bedroom.... is.... finished.

Eight hours of dusting, washing, sorting, tossing out. GADS we are packrats...

Two large trash bags for Goodwill of clothes we will never wear again, and FIVE feed sacks of trash—old magazines and catalogs mostly.

Got the guinea pigs cleaned and the living room done as well.

That only (?) leaves me with four rooms for tomorrow morning, then work, then shopping, then packing, then leaving.

By 3pm.

06 July 2007 at 12:15am

Well, we're here.

I got the four rooms to where they aren't a complete mess anymore, so when my friend comes to do the 'refresh' cleaning, all she'll have to do is vacuum the floors.

Took four hours.

We left out about quarter till five, but made excellent time in spite of the rain.

The good news is that we got our same suite at the hotel.

The bad news is that the a/c unit is blowing hot air. Rather than move, we got the windows open and they will fix it tomorrow.

Good thing we're not used to having a/c and that these windows actually open, huh?

06 July 2007 at 9:06pm

Bleck.

So.

12 hours later...

Got to the hospital and the appointments that showed on our computer were all different from the ones on the printout THEY gave us. Theirs completely deleted the pre-op with his surgeon and the blood work. Ward was all for this—said, "I'm sure they know what they are doing, Dear," and the only surly person we've met at MDA was at the reception desk and said the schedule was right. But Ward's mean old wife did some squawking and came to find out that it was computer error—the doctor had an emergency surgery this morning and told the schedulers to reschedule his early appointments and somehow Ward's got dropped altogether—and if I hadn't squawked, he couldn't have had his surgery on Monday.

But that took 3 hours to get resolved.

Which pushed everything ELSE back.

But we got 'er done:

-Surgeon says it's a go.
-Cardiologist says it's a go.
-Anesthesiologist says it's a go.

So we'll be at the hospital bright and early (5:15am check in) Monday morning.

In between appointments, I ran to the cafeteria and got Alec lunch and delivered it to the kids' room.

Then we went shopping for provisions, picked up the dog, and came back to the hotel.

Made some dinner (and splurged on French Silk pie for dessert), Ward and Alec are doing Alec's schoolwork and then to BED—we got about 4 hours sleep last night.

Wheeeeeeeee...

09 July 2007 at 12:31am

Check in is 5:15, surgery scheduled to begin at 7.

Estimated time in surgery between 8 and 10 hours.

Then at least an hour in recovery.

Then at least 24 hours in ICU.

Then we'll see...

10 July 2007 at 9:03pm

You know what I hate?

I hate when they tell you your loved one will be in ICU for at least 48 hours and when you call they say, "No change- he's doing fine but pretty out of it." And then you show up like an HOUR later you approach the room in ICU and see

an empty bed.

I hate that.

He's doing well enough that they moved him to a regular room in less than 24 hours, and he was sitting up eating soup when we left him 2 hours ago.

I told Alec in detail what all the surgery sites looked like and gave him the option of going to see him.... or not. Of course he said, "I WANNA SEE MY DAD." Upon inspecting the skin graft over the eye (which is very swollen to the point of being creased down the middle, and though it's warm and has normal color is obviously NOT face skin) he said, "Looks like he's got a tongue on the side of his face."

Between that and the Frankenstonian zipper scar all along his head, Ward is pretty excited about his new look.

PS—there is nothing cuter than a really serious, quiet dude on Free Access Morphine...

12 July 2007 at 10:27am

Well, Ward looked 100% better yesterday. The swelling is going down and they took all his IV lines out (including the little green button—THAT depressed him...), and he was a lot more lucid as well (hmmmm, something to do WITH the little green button???) He is eating off the menu and taking forced walks around the floor. The nurse showed us how to empty the drains (ew)—he has one on his arm and one on his head—and then we also got directions for incision care.

I have GOT to figure something out so he can see—he cannot wear his glasses because the sidepiece would rub his graft.

Wonder how long it would take an optical place to do up a monocle?

Today we have ordered a wheelchair and have an appointment to get his hair washed and then something to keep it tidy since the ponytail thing just doesn't hold up in bed. We're thinking cornrows...

15 July 2007 at 6:13pm

We've had a rough few days.

After doing so well, Ward took a nosedive (looked literal) on Thursday and had A LOT of swelling on his head/neck. Everything turned purple and his one remaining eye practically swole shut. They couldn't get the stupid leg wound to stop bleeding, and the graft on his head BLISTERED (height of ICKY). This was accompanied by A LOT of pain, and my normally even-tempered, perfect, patient husband got ...testy.

Friday night, the nurse made sure they had my phone numbers written down "in case they needed to contact me and he was non-communicative."

They have finally gotten the swelling down, and the leg wound has slowed to seeping ooze. He never spiked a fever and never lost circulation in the head graft, so they just filled him with morphine and sat tight.

Well, today he's still pretty purple, and the blisters haven't quite all gone away, but he feels a lot better. The doctor said that where he normally would've sent him home tomorrow, because of these "odd" (his word) developments, he is keeping him an extra few days.

So we are looking at home by NEXT weekend. As much as we all want to go home, I know that the prudent thing to do is the conservative thing, because with it being a five hour drive, we can't just "run him back to the hospital" if something goes wrong.

I need pie.

Dang.

That's what we forgot at the store....

We did pick up some lovely long scarves for him—his surgery site is about 8" diagonally and a patch a) wouldn't cover it and b) would be too constricting as it heals.

It's looking more and more like 'pirate' is a viable career option for him...

15 July 2007 at 10:15pm

Blisters.

Now he's got blisters.

He got the blisters the day after the swelling, and that's when they started the Lasix to get rid of the swelling.

The only thing I could find on the 'net about blisters and grafts (that aren't burn grafts) is that one of the only causes is Furosemide therapy.

.... Bingo?

17 July 2007 at 11:11pm

As I survey our hotel room, I see the dog, the boy, and the HUSBAND.

Headed home tomorrow and we don't have to see MDA again till all the way the 30th when he comes back to get stitches out and dressing off of the leg (which is still oozing, dang it).

He got his hair washed and a nice sponge bath before we left the hospital. We have to get an appointment with his regular cardiologist ASAP when we get home, and he will probably take Ward off of Lovenox (injectable blood-thinner). Right now they have him on Lovenox AND Coumadin—no bleeding issues THERE.

So we will be on the road at 11am tomorrow and

home

by

suppertime.

18 July 2007 at 10:07pm

It's so quiet.
No ambulances.
No trucks.
No noisy wall-mounted temperature control unit.

Just the whisper of the fans
and the chirp of the crickets
and the cozy wrapping of our familiar old home.

We came back to happy animals thanks to our neighbor Patsy,
clean guinea pigs thanks to my friend Rebecca,
a clean house thanks to my friend Kellie,
a little money left in our pockets thanks to my friends at work,
and
a lasagna dinner thanks to our friends Jennifer and Bobby.

After two weeks, we returned with a weary and bruised, but
recovering, Ward thanks to the doctors and staff at MDA and, just
as importantly, thanks to the powerful energy directed at us from
literally all over the planet.

While Ward put his feet up and Alec caught up on his computer
deprivation, I snuck over to the new property (it was KIND of on
the way to get milk...) where it's even MORE quiet.

The birds were singing.
The creek was burbling.
The setting sun turned bazillion kinds of wildflowers in the
meadows into dancing Technicolor fairies.

In our sorry wreck of a garden spot was
one
perfect
tomato.

Well, of course I shared it with the boys. It was still warm from the
sunshine and very, very yumlicious.

I feel better.

20 July 2007 at 10:38am

Keeping fingers crossed today.

I HOPE that today's blood test will show that I can stop giving
Ward the Lovenox injections. I'm running out of spots on his
tummy that aren't already purple from them.

24 July 2007 at 10:37pm

Our appointments for next week are (so far):

-The plastic surgeon for stitches out and exam
-The cancer surgeon for exam and
-A CAT scan of his chest to see what all is up with the spot on his
lung that showed up on his head/neck CAT scan before surgery.

Have I used up all my prayers yet?

25 July 2007 at 11:16pm

So when I went out to our new place last week, I couldn't get the padlock to lock and I left it just "looking" locked. Not a big worry around here. I bought a new "contractor grade" lock and tonight after work we made a detour out there to change it out. It was the first time we've all been out there in almost a month. When we got out of the car, a pair of what looked for all the world to be falcons flew over our heads, calling.

We thought, "How cool is THAT? How often do you see a pair of falcons???"

Apparently, you see them constantly if they are keeping an eye on you.

Everywhere we went, the birds followed, perching well within view when we stopped somewhere. Sometimes we could see only one, but they called back and forth to each other.

My guess is that they have a nest somewhere on our place.

When we got home, we started looking up falcons (these are smaller than hawks, but bigger than kestrels) and I *think* we have Prairie Falcons. I'm going back in the morning with my camera(s) to get something concrete to compare to the photos I found.

On the one hand we are thinking how very special it would be to have these raptors nesting on our place.

Of course, with OUR luck, the DNR will swoop in and say "We're sorry—this is now a designated nesting area for these protected birds. You can't build anything here".

Added later: Our falcons are actually Mississippi Kites, and they are known for being very 'obvious' when they have young ones nearby. The confusing part was that I was seeing both the adults

*AND the juveniles. The adults are solid grey with black masks, and
the youngsters are brown/white speckled, like Prairie Falcons.*

We're right on the edge of their territory, so it's still really cool.

30 July 2007 at 12:06am

We made it in spite of TWO, count them, TWO traffic snarls from
accidents on I-45—
It was storming on and off and kinda slipperish.

I'm headed to bed. We have to be up at 5:30am to make our early
appointment, then (if the weather holds) the zoo before Ward's
CAT scan at 4:30pm.

We're thinking really hard, "It's only a shadow. It's only a
shadow.... It is NOT a tumor. It is NOT a tumor..."

31 July 2007 at 10:00pm

We left the hospital at 12:30pm, the hotel at 1:30pm, the HOUR
LONG traffic jam at 4:30pm, and just got home at 7:30pm to
unload the car, feed the boys, and start the wash so I'm not behind
as soon as I get up tomorrow.

I'm really too old for this.

Plastic surgeon took out all stitches and dressings and pronounced
him able to shower. HOORAY! He said the leg was completely
healed, the arm is sort of healed but doing about as it should, so
he's to leave it uncovered as much as possible, and the eye area is

not as far along as he thought it would be (still some swelling, a big scab where the blisters were, and it's turned an interesting elephant skin color and texture- but it's warm and the Doppler showed that it's still circulating up a storm, so he's just gonna see what happens there...)

Cancer doctor said that the CAT scan was inconclusive, and there ARE several "small areas" that *could* be scar tissue from some sort of lung infection in the past, or could be cancer. They want to do a PET scan, which is much more specialized and done in the Nuclear Medicine Area—thus needing special insurance approval and appointmentation. Soonest we could get in there is the 22nd. Which works, cuz that's when his two surgeons want to see him for another re-check anyway. That should tell us exactly what's going on in there.

Oh yeah. And they are also doing an ultrasound of his abdomen since the bottom edge of the chest CAT scan showed masses on his kidney and spleen.

Now.

We were told that it COULD have been those organs sucking up the CAT scan juice weird, and since they were not focusing on that area, it could just look 'funny,' but they want an ultrasound just to be sure.

We were told that for basal cell to jump to the lungs, kidney and spleen would be very, very rare. And that to have TWO primary cancers of different sorts (the jumping kind and the non-jumping kind) would be very, very, VERY rare.

We are all just about as frazzled as 3 people (and one old terrier) can be without coming completely unraveled.

So it's off to MDA again Tuesday night the 21st for appointments, and tests the 22nd, 23rd, 24th and we'll go from there.

Again.

Some more.
Bleah.

03 August 2007 at 12:30pm

Ok.
The cancer doctor we saw this week was the associate and she's the one who said "PET scan of the lungs and ultrasound of the abdomen."

I noticed that on the appointment calendar on the MDAnderson website he has only the PET scan scheduled.

I called the nurse and she said that Dr. Hanna (our primary doctor) came back into the office last night, saw what they found on the CAT scan and said, "We are DONE messing with this," and ordered the PET scan to be done of his entire body. That will show any cancer cells anywhere from the top of his head down to his knees. We'll know what's where and what we need to do about it.

I love Dr. Hanna.

07 August 2007 at 11:29am

Ward's been trying to go back to work some and now we think he's used his arm too much.

The most fragile part, dead center on the surgical site where the tendon was exposed, looks weepy and open and is a very unattractive yellow (though not oozy and it actually started out kinda light yellow).

They told us to leave it all exposed to dry and heal, but I've antibiotic-creamed that section, covered it with the Vaseline impregnated gauze dressing, and then with the ace bandage again.

I'm sending an email (with a pretty picture attached) to the doctor to see if we need to do anything else with it.

I sure hope it's something we can do from HERE; it's been really nice being at home.

07 August 2007 at 1:14pm

I understand keeping Ward in a clean environment is important.

Hmmmm, which clean environment shall we choose?

Our house with the winders open to the dust from the road on one side and the dust from the goat pen on the other side and the dogs and cats running around everywhere?

Or his work environment in the auto parts warehouse?

He's doomed....

I did get an email back from the PA (dang, they are fast down there...) and she said just a wet gauze pad with saline solution wrinkled on top of the affected area, then the loose bandage.

He's gonna be very excited when I tell him the cure is to put salt into his open wound.

20 August 2007 at 11:31pm

Headed back down yonder tomorrow afternoon...

We've got the plastic surgeon recheck on Wednesday, tests
Wednesday and Thursday, and on Friday…

the cancer doctor who will tell us which way our lives will be
going...

21 August 2007 at 2:21pm

Today:

-Did laundry and hung it out.

-Spent half of the morning on the phone shuffling appointments
down yonder. Up till last Friday, we had all Thursday open and
promised Alec we'd go to NASA. Then BANG—an ultrasound
scheduled for 1pm Thursday. They managed to shift it to tomorrow
morning before our other appointments.

-Spent the other half making sure work is all set for the next few
weeks as far as scheduling, supplies, and whatnot, and all our bills
are caught up and pre-paid.

-Spent the OTHER other half cleaning the guinea pigs.

-Took showers.

-Eating lunch now.

NOW we need to:

-Go to the bank
-The feed store
-The grocery store
-The drug store
-Wash the car
-Come home and
-Pack our clothes
-Food
-Toys/books/etc.
Into the car and leave by 3pm.

What are our chances?

21 August 2007 at 10:56pm

Nope. Didn't leave at 3pm, but we DID leave at a respectable 4:08pm.

Back in Houston now. Yik.

Alec is running amok with a boy from down the way here—running running running running...

Hope it helps him sleep after the 5-hour drive.

22 August 2007 at 5:10pm

Kidney and spleen look excruciatingly normal according to the radiologist. Ward's in getting his PET scan now. Then to the GROCERY STORE—he hasn't been able to eat since 7:30 this morning.

Cancer doctor is Friday at noon.

Tomorrow we are going to NASA- Alec's request.

We are ALL relieved—our attitudes have improved 357% since this morning.

Oh.

And our 'regular' economy sized suite hotel room was taken by a patient who needed to extend their stay, so we got an upgrade—bedroom w/bath and TV, living room with sleeper sofa/bath/TV and kitchen. Normally $199 per night, for the lower rate we booked at.

24 August 2007 at 4:25pm

Normal

Perfectly, wonderfully freakin' ***normal*** from the tip of his dear pointy head to the bottoms of his sexy manly feets—he's cancer-free, cancer-less, sans cancer.

They want us to see a radiation doctor to discuss whether or not they want to do any radiation "just in case," and we have regular post surgical rechecks in 8 weeks.
But as far as we are concerned,

We may now resume our regularly scheduled lives.

12 September 2007 at 7:39pm

Well crap.

The radiologist called this afternoon saying that after reviewing last year's records YES HE DOES want to follow-up this latest surgery with another course of radiation.

That means 7 weeks in Houston—a week to set it all up and 6 weeks of getting zapped every day.

Consecutively.

So about three grand for the cheap hotel alone.
Plus food.
Plus gas.

And Ward probably losing his job cuz that's a long time for them to go without an inventory manager.

So that means no more insurance.

And him being down there alone cuz *I* can't be away from MY job that long.

...Now what?

12 September 2007 at 9:27pm

Here's what my gut feeling says:

-The PET scan says there's no cancer. It's pretty darn accurate.

I want to talk to the plastic surgeon to see what 6 weeks of radiation will do to his brand-new, beautifully alive graft that they mutilated his arm to get.

I want to talk to the cancer surgeon to see how often they are gonna PET scan him anyway. Cuz if we have all healthy tissue NOW, why would we want to burn it all up???
And if they are gonna PET scan him like every 3 months, couldn't we jump on the radiation wagon if/when we SEE cancer again and they have something to AIM at rather than just shot gunning his head???

I understand that "since this was/is a very aggressive cancer we want to treat aggressively so it doesn't come back—therefore we feel it would be beneficial at this time to irradiate the area,"

(Little voice in my head) BUT THERE'S NO CANCER THERE— WHAT ARE YOU KILLING????

15 September 2007 at 1:05am

Interesting day.

Picked up the pathology report from after his surgery last year. You know, the one where they said the pathology report came back negative so they sewed him up? Well the INITIAL pathology report the day of surgery did come back negative.

Here's what the FINAL report says:

"Sections demonstrate residual basal cell carcinoma present. Tumor measures 2.0cm in greatest dimensions. The lateral inferior and lateral superior soft tissue margins are positive for tumor."

And I was so hoping that it was a clerical mishap and someone filed the final report without the doctor seeing/knowing about it, but it says here:

"The findings were discussed with Dr. ****** on 5/15/06.
(Signed) *******, MD Pathologist"

Four days. That was four days post-op.
He was still in the hospital.
She could have gone back in to get it.

But she didn't.

I am beyond pissed.

The correspondence from the radiologist to the surgeon clearly states that they KNEW there was still cancer. But they never told us. They didn't do a scan before radiation to make sure they were even AIMING at the right spot and SURPRISE SURPRISE, less than a year later the cancer was back and we got to go through this past summer of more surgery/testing/scanning/mutilation (both the cancer site and the donor sites for the NEW graft).

His very first surgery for this cancer was 5 years ago—they did Mohs microsurgery and NO radiation. Took it 4 years to become problematic again. I'm not convinced that the radiation didn't make the area more favorable for cancer growth.

So that's why we're a little twitchy about more radiation. Especially since their PET scan says there's NO CANCER THERE.

But that's not the point.

The POINT is that THIS past summer could have been avoided.

Last summer.

When she got back the final report she could have:

-Gone back to surgery

-Sent him to a CANCER surgeon (she's an eye surgeon)

-Sent him directly to MDAnderson.

We would not have thought less of her for saying, "You know, this thing is a bear, and I think it's out of my level of knowledge so I'm referring you to Dr. X".

But I can't form words for what I think of her now.

15 September 2007 at 5:01pm

We have an appointment Tuesday to talk to an attorney recommended by the referral service that the American Cancer Society gave me.

I don't WANNA go there.

But dang it—NO family should have to go through what we are going through just because some doctor wanted to look omnipotent.

My tummy hurts.

We don't want punishment per se, or revenge, or an eye for an eye (hmmmm....).

Just something that will make her do the RIGHT thing in the future.

I'm a non-drinker, but I AM fixin' to mix up a root beer float and head to bed—Alec is watching a lovely documentary about killer ants.

20 September 2007 11:53pm

I just want Ward to be well, and for all the bullshit to cease.

No more tests,

No more doctors,

No more travels or expenses.

Just a normal, boring life.

22 September 2007 at 7:45pm

The LAST course of radiation was *every day* for six weeks, and it left a big ol' tumor intact.

We'd love to discuss with the doctor how he got from "we probably won't" to "oh, let's do," but I am getting the royal run around from the radiation staff at MDA. Apparently the patient is supposed to accept "because I'm the Doctor and I said so" and then eagerly sign up to be radiated.

Not thinking so.

I've talked to nurses, PA's, and schedulers, and left messages (?!) for our assigned Patient Advocate, and gotten everything from, "We have to talk to the doctor- a SECOND consult is not usually done" (HELLOOOO? he didn't have the records in front of him to do a proper consult on the FIRST visit), to a flat out, "We realize you have to do what's best for your family, but YOU need to decide which is more important—your husband's health, or being inconvenienced" (referring to Ward's job loss due to being away for six weeks and resultant loss of insurance). Boy THAT chick has MY vote for Customer Service Angel of the Month.

We just want to sit down in the same room with the freakin' doctor and get his reasons for wanting to do this so we can make an informed decision.

Unreasonable????

Meanwhile....

The lawyer took all the info and will go over it with his medical person.

IF the treatment he received would have been the same with or without RETAINED TUMOR, even though it was clearly bad judgment to not tell the PATIENT about the CANCER that she left in his body, it's questionable as to whether or not it would be negligence.

Of course, there's the other end of the radiation where he was released (in writing) back into her care and she did no post-radiation scans.

You know. To be sure it was gone.

Of course we never questioned it, because we thought there was NOTHING THERE to begin with.

My head hurts.

I've taken drugs and I'm going to bed.

24 September 2007 1:16am

We have to go back to Houston tomorrow.

Tomorrow.

Not next week.

Tomorrow.

I hate it with a heat that rivals the sun.

Nay, a million suns.

Crap.

25 September 2007 at 12:52am

Our good news today—finally talked to the Radiologist Oncologist. His staff WAS running interference and he just got my message (one of like a hundred in the last TWO WEEKS). Apparently I was given PART of his evaluation. The message SHOULD have been relayed thusly:

"A further course of radiation MAY be of benefit, BUT considering the time since surgery, the fact that it's resisted past radiation given in the same time frame (three months post op), the distance that the patient lives from the facility, and resultant hardships radiation would most likely cause, I feel that as long as we follow closely as the surgeon is planning with frequent scans, I'd just as soon save the 'silver bullet' of radiation for when/if recurrent cancer is detected and removed—starting radiation as soon as possible after surgery."

I made sure that the doctor was aware of the difficulty I had getting through to him, while thanking him profusely for calling us personally.

As an aside, Ward's plastic surgeon from last year (good doctor— the one who found the cancer this time) called the house this evening to see if we'd heard from the radiologist and when I told him the trouble I'd had he told me, "If it's any consolation, I tried calling him today and *I* couldn't get through to him, either". Dang.

Bad news (maybe) is that Ward's orbital graft started leaking clear stuff yesterday, so I sent a photo to the plastic surgeon this morning telling them that it doesn't hurt, isn't discolored or odiferous, and he's not running fever. And that we will be down yonder next Wednesday anyhow for another consult, so could stop to see him then.

Within 30 minutes, they had us set up for an appt THIS Wednesday.

Fabulous.

So I thought I had all week to prepare for being gone NEXT week, and now I have...today.

And I have to prepare as if we will be gone longer than 2 days since historically with him being diabetic, infection = hospitalization w/IV antibiotics. Double fabulous.

Other bad news was that the lawyer got back to us and declined the case. Said that with the new caps on awards, he can only afford to take those that he called 'jaw droppers'—where the jury hears what happened and faints clear away. Specifically, those cases that result in death.

So since Ward is selfishly still alive, it's not a big enough case.

He said (and I can see this) that with it being cancer, it would be impossible to prove that, even if the original doctor had treated it differently, it wouldn't have come back.

So even though his medical expert wholeheartedly agreed that she should have told us about the remaining cancer and given us options, it's not provable negligence or malpractice.

My mantra for the next XX,XXX,XXX days is:

"No radiation is good. Deal with the rest as it comes".

25 September 2007 at 11:37pm

We're here in Houston now, and are going to try to see our NEXT week's doctor tomorrow so we won't have to come back till mid-month.

And, apparently, in-between work, errands, laundry, and packing this morning, I bought a truck.

I can hardly wait to go home to meet it.

27 September 2007 at 12:46am

The stupid TV went out in the hotel last night. The boys cannot survive without one, so we had to move all our stuff for one stinkin' night.

At the new room the Internet didn't work.

Ward's all pissy and I don't know why.

I'm happy that he's OK—just a mild sinusitis— and we're all excited about the new truck, but DANG, I'm tired.

Because it's like, 1am.

28 September 2007 at 12:27pm

The update on Ward's infection: as yakky as it is to imagine the goop from sinusitis settling behind the graft via the hole still there to the sinus cavity and then oooooooozing out, it's still better than the graft itself being infected.

Way, way, way better.

We did get a chance to see the nurse and nutritionist for the Palliative Care doctor and did the first half of our appointment. Couldn't see the doctor as he refuses to overbook (a good thing since that means he takes A LOT of time with EVERYONE). I liked the nurse immediately. She has a wedding ring that looks like it was made by the same jeweler as mine—astounding because these rings were made in the '30's and I've never seen one as similar. Mine has sapphires and hers has emeralds, and the design is very slightly different, but you have to set them side by side to see any difference. As a big fan of antique jewelry, I took this as a very good sign.

But more importantly, in looks and manner she reminded both of us A LOT of our friend Cheryl, which is a VERY good sign.

We took home the questionnaires that we need to fill out for the doctor for when we see him and were able to move that appointment to the day before Ward's surgical recheck, so we don't have to go down there again for THREE WHOLE WEEKS.

On the way home we stopped at a Whole Earth Store (cool but pretty spendy), and a Bookstop that's in a renovated old movie house (WAY cool) and stopped for lunch at the Sam Houston Visitors' Center to see up close and personal the statue we've passed a dozen gazillion times this summer.

So overall, a pretty good trip, even though unexpected.

I called the car dealership and he's gonna call me when my truck is ready—I had told them there was no rush as we didn't know when we'd be home.

So maybe later today...

2 October 2007 at 10:50pm

It's official.

I have IBS.

Doctor says I've been borderline for several years and this summer's combo of stress and travel pushed me right over the edge.

So I really AM full of it.

I get new drugs tomorrow so we'll see if that helps. I'm sick of tummy troubles.

Of course, "just to be sure," I also have to provide a sample.

Perfect.

10 October 2007 11:09pm

We don't qualify for any money or help or special programs or anything for medical bills OR the new farm.

We make just enough money to be disqualified for all the above, and not enough to actually pay for any of it.

Bleah.

22 October 2007 at 1:16am

Houston, we have a problem.

Literally.

Just got back tonight, and have to head back yonder tomorrow.

I really
Really
Really
Really   .
Really
REALLY
Hate this....

25 October 2007 at 9:58am

-Plastic surgeon says more surgery, a little more extensive than the other surgeon thought—more openings and cuttings and possibly drain tubes and whatnot.

-We go see the cardiologist in an hour to see what he wants to do about the Coumadin issue—I hope no Lovenox again...

-Back here to MDA Tuesday so we can see the anesthesiologist bright and early Wednesday morning, then surgery early Thursday morning. (So no Halloween party for us. No Halloween at all because I'm so NOT trick or treating in stupid HOUSTON).

They will keep him in hospital for a few days after surgery, so hopefully home by next Sunday night. Then, of course, rechecks, tubes out, sutures out, etc, etc, etc, frequently till it's all healed up.

They've scheduled his next PET scan for the week between Christmas and New Year's, the earliest appointment in the time frame the surgeon wanted, which means NO vacation for us then, which is kind of a moot point, since after this little bit we'll have less than no money for that anyway, and if we request that they do it later, we'll be into a whole new year for the insurance, meaning we'll have to pay for all of it.

I know I'm whining, and I know it could be so much worse—the cancer back or somewhere else, bigger heart issues, all sorts of stuff, and that in the grand scheme of things this is just an annoyance, but dammit, Alec was really into the Halloween party stuff, made and sent invitations, did all the planning, all of it.

And he hasn't seen his brother and sister since LAST summer—they didn't make it last Christmas, and this past summer's vacation was put off till THIS Christmas due to us being down here with the original surgery.

Poor little guy is trying really hard not to be outwardly sad about it all, but it's hard for ME—I can't imagine what's going on in his 7-year-old mind.

And of course Ward thinks he's ruined all our lives.

25 October 2007 at 8:12pm

We're back.

Cardiologist visit went really, really well—said to stop taking the Coumadin immediately and NO Lovenox (woo hoo!)

Tomorrow I'll sit down with the bills and juggle 'em all around yet again, make some phone calls, beg for mercy...so far I've been able to make it work, I'll just have to keep doing it.

Most of the time creditors are pretty good about stuff if you call and talk to them, I just thought after doing that this whole summer, I could finally see the light at the end of the tunnel.

But it was just the headlight of another stupid train.

...Whining again—guess I'll go make the boys some supper.

One good thing—as long as we've got chickens, we've always got eggs.

31 October 2007 at 2:20pm

We met with the anesthesiologist this morning and got all our blood work and pre-registration done.

Also dropped poor Spooj at the kennel till tomorrow after we're done at the hospital.

Now we just need to call the hospital between 3pm-5pm today to get our report time for in the morning.

I am somewhat bothered that what started out as "a little repair work" is scheduled in for a FIVE-HOUR SURGERY, including a possible wound vac drain, which would need ANOTHER surgery to remove.

Drat.

Nice day, anyway—Ward's taking a little nap, and then we're headed out to the museum district.

31 October 2007 at 6:28pm

We have to be at the hospital at 5:15 tomorrow morning.

Alec just informed me he has a sore throat.

How the heck will I be two places at once????

I can't fudge and say Alec's fine if he's not—and bring a germy kid into an environment of all immune-suppressed people.

And I can't just dump Ward off at the curb.

Shit.

31 October 2007 at 10:01pm

No fever yet. We've had dinner and Alec's had his shower, so I'm drugging him up good with Children's' Advil Cold and Flu, and trying to get Mr. Night Owl to go to sleep early.

LAST surgery I had my friend Cathy here.

This time, no one to stay with Alec if he needs to stay at the hotel.

...Figures.

01 November 2007 at 6:27pm

Alec so far is holding tough, so that's positive.

We got to the hospital at 5:15am and they took Ward back at 7am. He was in recovery, sitting up watching TV at 11am and in a room by noon. No swelling at all. Looking great. We were happy and optimistic about going home over the weekend.

Fools

Then the doctor came in.

-He wants to keep Ward till at least early next week so they can get him back on blood thinners for his clotting issues, and keep the stitches AND the drain in for "a long time" so his thinned blood does not do what he thinks happened last time (see below).
-From what he saw during surgery, what he thought was tissue swelling after the first surgery was more likely the socket filling with his nice thin blood and pushing the graft forward. That blood then kinda sat there (ick) and finally started oozing out the edges (double ick).

-Of course Ward needs to be on some sort of thinner so his annoying cardiac clots don't come back, so the doctor is not completely convinced that it won't happen again and we'll lose the graft, which can't be re-done since he's already used all the parts needed for one.
-He mentioned the use of therapeutic leeches.

-Oh. And by the way, he's leaving for Japan tomorrow night.

So tomorrow I need to sit outside the cardiologist's office till they can see me and tell me what they are planning to put him on since the Coumadin was causing him to break out in hives for the last month.

They said that was not a side effect of Coumadin (in very condescending voices), but dang if 12 hours after going off Coumadin he was completely freakin' healed—not an itch or even a light bruise left, and he had been positively purple all over from scratching.

I think we'll be ordering pizza delivered tonight.

If there is a God, they will also deliver cheesecake.

02 November 2007 at 11:14pm

Alec sorta crashed and burned today—very snurfly and a headache and that *sick* look in his eyes. So we went to the Kroger's to get cold medicine and new markers and a new drawing book and he's been drugged and quiet all day—the only time we went out other than to the store was to sit at the picnic table in the sun to do his schoolwork.

He seems better tonight, still sniffly but not snurfly, and he didn't ever have a fever, so unless he takes a turn for the worse, we'll be able to go up to see Ward tomorrow.

Speaking of Ward, I raised some Cain with the cardio department today. They said that he's not technically a patient of theirs, so he is not assigned a set doctor. Whoever is making rounds is seeing him—which led to one of those doctors giving him a Lovenox injection LAST NIGHT when his chart states that the surgeon wants NO blood thinners for at least 48 hours after surgery, and then a very gradual re-starting of them over several more days.

Guess what? He now has an assigned doctor, and they are working up a plan for him so he gets just enough thinner to keep him from forming clots, but not enough to pool blood behind his graft again.

Wow.

Wish *I* had thought of that.

I also called his cardiologist in Tyler to tell him what's going on and to express our desire for something OTHER than Coumadin for the long term.

Ward did get the following info from his surgeon:

-He's only gone to Japan for the weekend.

-He wants to leave the drain in at least two weeks, when we'll see him for the first re-check.

The TSU/Southern University college game is tomorrow at the Astrodome (right across the street from our hotel), making our parking lot Party Central tonight.

We didn't get cheesecake, but we DID get a pint of Extreme Moose Tracks ice cream for Alec and a pint of Caramel Sutra ice cream for mommy.

03 November 2007 at 9:32am

The football partiers were pretty well-behaved last night—a few loud conversations, some breakage of bottles, and a LOT of boom box type music. We'll see what tonight brings.

Guess it depends on who wins the game...

Ward was concerned for us, but I told him it's not "those crazy college kids," it's mostly families—so I guess the relatives of the players and alumni?

Alec seems better this morning, so we'll head out in a bit to go see Ward—doggy daycare is only open till 3pm today.

Then back here to do laundry.

Woo hoo.

04 November 2007 at 12:05pm

I talked on the phone with the cardiologist doing rounds today, and boy howdy is he lucky I wasn't in the room with him. He'd a had his ears boxed for sure.
I wanted to talk with him so they could think of something OTHER than Coumadin to put Ward on—he's supposed to start up again tomorrow.

First he tried to explain to me why they took him off before surgery (DUH). Second, he told me they hadn't restarted it yet because he has a dental procedure scheduled for tomorrow (WHAT??????) Then he told me that the hives coulda been caused by any of Ward's other meds.

I tried to tell him nicely that none of his other meds had been changed and all the symptoms were GONE within 12 hours of going off Coumadin which, in my totally unprofessional opinion was PRETTY DANG INDICATIVE. Then he said that they could always just try aspirin if Ward couldn't tolerate the Coumadin, but HE couldn't do it- that was the surgeon's call.

I told him that the surgeon had told us it was CARDIO'S call.

Then he said it was really his long-term home-based cardiologist's call to make any changes to medication, and if he reacted badly to the Coumadin again that our Tyler guy would be making the changes.

I pointed out that the cardio guys (HIS department) at MDA had already taken Ward off of Cordorone and onto a beta-blocker, so apparently they CAN make those decisions, and don't we think Ward's been through enough without having to be HIVISH again before trying a different blood thinner???

He finally said he'd be talking to the other department doctors and the surgery guys and they'd come up with something.

When I talked to Ward later he asked me why the heart doctor was crying after talking on the phone to me (I don't think he really was—Ward was just trying to cheer me up).

He also told me that the doctor admitted that it was a whole DIFFERENT PATIENT getting dental work tomorrow.

He got on the phone with a family member looking at the WRONG DANG CHART.

Today is beauteous, and we're headed to the park. Spooj's daycare is only available from 4-6pm, so that's when we'll go see Ward.

04 November 2007 at 12:32pm

What really gets my goat is that these guys are all so specialized that they can't/won't see past their own little parts of the body. Now, if you have a patient with only one problem at hand, that's fine. But if you have, say, a patient with cancer, heart issues, AND diabetes (Hey look—here's one—wave "hello," Mr. Dixon...) they all have to work TOGETHER, dang it, or the surgeon does stuff that endangers the heart, and the heart guy does stuff to endanger the surgery healing.

I KNOW they have to keep his blood thin, cuz if he develops a clot in his heart that doesn't get caught/dissolved in a timely manner, it could break loose and kill him.

I KNOW they have to keep his blood thick, cuz if it pools behind his graft again and the graft fails, he'll be stuck with just a socket again.

I KNOW if he's stuck with just a socket again, healing will be slow, or impossible, cuz the head is an extremity and he's got diabetes. And if it never heals, eventually he'll get an infection, which could kill him.

But SURELY, in the BEST CANCER HOSPITAL IN THE WORLD, SOMEONE will be able to figure it out, and it'd be nice if they could do it without little Mrs. Barely Made It Through High School having to lead them by the hand.

End rant (for now).

I am well aware that a lot of the time, they listen to me and make changes just to shut me up.

And I'm OK with that.

04 November 2007 at 7:20pm

What a lovely afternoon at the park—sun shining, birds singing, happy families, a band playing in the band shell, roses blooming, yada, yada, yada.

Dropped Spooj off at daycare, went up to the hospital, picked up a snack, and headed to the 11th floor.

Hmmm.

Curious.

A big STOP sign on Ward's door. Instructions to don protective gown and gloves before entering.

NOW WHAT???

Apparently, his cultures have come back positive for MRSA. A superbug. Great.

A cursory search on the 'net got me this info:

-There's a good chance he got it there in the hospital.

-Patients who acquire MRSA have three times the length of hospital stays (14 days as opposed to 4), rack up twice the hospital bill, and have a lovely 11% chance of never making it out of the hospital at all.

-It's been found that diabetic patients recover much more quickly when the super-antibiotics (which he is getting via IV) are accompanied by

Maggot therapy.

CAN TODAY *GET* ANY BETTER?????

08 November 2007 at 9:20pm

He's OUT.
Finally OUT.
We got him all released this afternoon and are headed back
tomorrow.

Of course we can't go HOME—he has to see his local cardiologist
at 3:30pm for lab work, and THEN we can go home.

Till next week.
But we don't know when.
They'll let us know.
Sometime next week.

Have they ever tried to make work and lodging arrangements using
'sometime next week' as time parameters?

Weasels.

At least I still have my sunny disposition.

14 November 2007 at 9:43pm

OK

Gone and back home already.

-Doctor took out the drain tube, but said he wants to leave the
stitches in another few weeks, so we go back on the 5th for that.

-He's still on the oral antibiotics so they didn't culture for the
MRSA yet.

Even though we had a 10am appointment and we didn't see the doctor till ELEVEN THIRTY, we were still able to have a picnic in the Japanese Garden in the museum district and then make our way home.

We're...so...happy...to...be...able...to...unpack...the...suitcases...

05 December 2007 at 11:50pm

And yet another "quickie: visit.

Ward got his sutures out today and the plastic surgeon said he does NOT want to see us back there for at LEAST six months.

They took another culture to see if it'll grow MRSA, but since there's no sign of infection, if it DOES show up, it'll just be a longer dose of oral antibiotics and more culturing.

We did meet up with a friend for a minute—she bought all my candle-making stuff and we brought them some eggs, and we got yummy pickles and some Watkins samples. We left them off at the museum and headed home...

...Where we can stay for TWO WHOLE WEEKS. Ward's first quarterly PET scan is on the 20th, and we find out the results on the 21st.

Dear Santa,
All I want for Christmas this year and forever is for my little family to be healthy and whole.
Thank you very much.
I do believe in you.
sheri

06 December 2007 at 12:09am

One more trip to Houston before Christmas.

This PET scan had better be positive in our favor, or I will go stark raving crazy insane mad.

It's time to get back to our lives.

Cancer has taken a big enough toll.

I so decree.

20 December 2007 at 9:26am

On the way down last night, Alec started complaining of a sore throat, and by 1am he had a fever, and by 5am he'd puked.

So now I've got coffee, and the boys are still sleeping.

Ward's scan is at 12:30, and he'll have to go alone.

I am hoping like all get-out that I can get this kid's fever down this morning and hold it down—he won't be allowed in hospital if he's had fever/sore throat/pukage 24 hours prior, and I do NOT want Ward going to the consult after the scan reading alone.

Just in case.

20 December 2007 at 1:14pm

Well, Alec tossed, turned, whimpered and fevered till well after 9am, so Ward left a little bit ago for his scan by himself.

I'm fixin' to make some soup for the little guy, who says his throat and head still hurt, but the fever is mostly under control, and he's had some yogurt and tea, and asked for some clothes so he could get dressed.

Now he's reading, so I'm tentatively optimistic that we'll be able to take him with us tomorrow.

21 December 2007 at 9:14pm

Whew

When we saw the doctor this morning, the doctor who did the MRI and the one who read it accompanied him. They said that although there's no indication of CANCER there, there was "something" that appeared to be an air pocket. Upon examination, we could clearly see the HOLE that was hiding under his last surgical scab that fell off this morning in the shower, but that has been allowing air to seep under the graft. It's about 1/8" in diameter, and perfectly round.

So.

They called the plastic surgeon, who dropped what he was doing and came up to the head and neck department and they all stared at it.

They decided to put a few stitches in it and hope for the best, although they are not very confident that it's gonna heal, meaning at some point in the next 6 months, they believe they will have to totally and completely re-do the graft. They will try to find a donor site (probably from his lower back for the main graft, then from his OTHER thigh for skin to cover it) and pull up another vessel from lower down on his neck and go farther out than the current edges. Between his diabetes and the fact that they irradiated that area last year, it's going to be a difficult road to complete healing.

Sigh.

So, instead of our hoped-for end of March scan, we go back in three weeks to have these stitches taken out, and again three weeks after that for a re-check and another MRI to see if the air pocket's gone.

We ARE happy.
We ARE grateful.
We WILL have a terrific Christmas.
This is just another bump in the road...
Or three.
Or seven.

I know I'm being just a big fat hairy whiner
Because I'm tired
And I'm stressed
And I'm basically just a big fat hairy whiner.

Alec is much improved- he drove us nuts all the way home, so we knew he felt better.

26 December 2007 at 12:00pm

Well, the stupid stitches that the doctor SAID wouldn't work have already come open. I KNEW they wouldn't hold. The tissue around the opening is BLACK, like *NOT viable*.

Ward is very discouraged and does NOT want to redo the whole graft surgery. I know nothing about people medicine and just a bit about animals, but I'd THINK that they could:

-Get an ear/nose/throat guy in to block that opening from his nasal cavity to behind the graft (it's where tear ducts would normally empty into, but helLO, his eye's gone- what are they afraid of? disfigurement???)

-Make sure that the back of the graft/front of the donor site is not all dried out from the air in there so they can heal together like they are supposed to.

-Trim the non-viable tissue so there are clean edges to pull together and THEN stitch it up after sucking all the air out from behind (maybe poofing some of that nice powdered antibiotic in there as well...)

-Apply a pressure bandage to hold that firmly in place no matter if he sneezes or snores or whatever during healing.

Whatever...

I'm taking pictures to email to the doctor this morning with our concerns and questions—he's got an EXCELLENT PA who looks at and answers emails promptly, and the doctor is always in the company of her and at least 2 or 3 other doctors/students (Ward calls 'em Dr. Hanasono's Posse) who he doesn't lord over, but consults with. I really can't see him as a "my way or the highway" kinda guy, but I guess we're fixin' to find out...

Hopefully we'll get some direction today—IF they all aren't out of pocket for the holidays.

Oh. And way back when, after the first surgery, when his arm was having trouble healing, I suggested we use a topical ointment called Facilitator. It's a vet product that promotes healing and discourages the formation of "proud flesh", or "granulation tissue" in horses, which is caused by normal tissue filling in a wound site too quickly and too exuberantly, causing a bumpy and abnormal area.

I actually have a friend who used it on herself (unbeknownst to her doctor) after a barrel horse flipped over on her and the saddle horn pretty much scalped her—she had to be life flighted to Dallas. They told her she'd need extensive plastic surgery to get rid of the scarring that'd come with healing. Using the Facilitator alone, you have to catch her face at just the right angle in just the right light to even see a line there.

Ward pooh poohed me, and we went back to Houston several times just to have the granulation tissue trimmed off, then the healing had to start over each time.

Last night, Ward was talking to his brother, the VET, and Mike suggested using the same dang thing and Ward told me, "Mike thinks this may work, can we get some?"

$%^&*(^! @#$%^$$#@#!!!!!!!!!!!!

And the answer is NO. We can't. MIKE hasn't even seen this. Ward needs to get the air OUT of there. He needs VIABLE tissue for it to adhere to or it won't close up. And if it DID close up with the air in there, he's setting himself up for a nice SEALED ABSCESS, which will blow the ENtire graft off of there, then kill him.

...Men.

27 December 2007 at 1:09pm

OK—we have an OFFICIAL appointment on Wednesday at 9am
with the plastic surgeon
so "all" I have to do is:

-Get payroll out the morning of the 1st and drive down yonder that afternoon.

-Situate the puppies so they don't completely tear down the house while we are gone. (Our Great Pyrenees had pups Thanksgiving week and they're big enough to make trouble, but not big enough to go outside yet- especially with no one home).

-Try to keep both boys germ-free (they are both still snurfling and sore-throaty).

I *think* we will just be seeing the doctor for getting a plan formed. Since Ward's still on Coumadin, I don't think he can just stuff him in hospital next week, so we *should* have till after most of the puppies are gone before we are in Houston for an extended stay.

Another extended stay.

Sigh.

2008

01 January 2008 at 10:49pm

We're here.

In our lovely hotel room.

In luxurious southwest Houston.

Our appointment is at 9am tomorrow and we WILL be going home straight afterwards.

This is just a "figure out what we'll be doing to fix the hole in his head and then schedule it for later" kind of trip.

...I can hear puppies gleefully tearing up my house from here...

02 January 2008 at 8:00pm

Ok.
The good news is that:

-The MRSA 2nd culture came back negative—one to go (they pulled one today) and he's officially safe to be in public.
-There's no infection at the site of the graft.
-The sun was shining today.

The bad news is:

-He has to have the whole graft replaced.

There are several reasons I did NOT kill the doctor-

#1—He had 2 other doctors with him and they'd just spent an hour going over Ward's chart, the CAT scans, the MRI's, and everything they could find on this sort of weird graftal behavior, trying to think of a way they could do exactly what I had posted here last week re: repairing without re-grafting.

#2—The main problem is that the air pocket is being caused not by a *hole*, but by more of a *sieve* area that's allowing air to leak, so it needs a good, fat graft literally stuffed in there and packed tight to seal it. His current graft is fully healed, but is too tight and too thin now to stretch down in there all the way.

#3—They said that when they do the next "procedure," they will take a big ol' honkin' hunk of muscle from his tummy or back and then close that with an incision, not leave it wide open like his poor arm, then take a skin graft from his leg to cover THAT on his head—so healing will be much easier, less ouchy, and much less prone to infection than the first time.

We have to go back anyway for another cancer-finding MRI the first week of Feb, and they have scheduled a detailed CAT scan so they can get their game plan for surgery at that time.

Then they'll bring him back a few weeks later for the actual surgery.

Meanwhile, we need to get his cardiologist to do another round of tests so they can take him off of Coumadin altogether before/during/immediately after surgery so there should be NO stupid blood leakage into that surgical area again.

I calmly but firmly informed them that as far as a surgery date, since Ward will be in hospital anywhere from 4-12 days, they have to plan around Alec's birthday on February 17th.

-We've had to cancel our family vacation TWICE because of being in the hospital.
-We spent Halloween in the hospital.
-We spent the days just prior to Christmas in the hospital.
-We were on our WAY to the hospital on New Years Day.
-There's no way they are fucking up this boy's birthday.

They said they understood.

And the fear in their eyes told me that they really, really did.

13 January 2008 at 11:34pm

We are perilously close to losing most everything we own and I have no stinking idea how we are going to afford this next go-around.

I don't even have money enough to pay the utilities this month.

I'm so proud of Ward and Alec for being so brave and pleasant through everything, and only wish I were half as gracious.

But I'm not.

17 January 2008 at 10:14pm

We have a schedule.

Feb 4th—bloodwork/xrays/CAT scans/MRI's

Feb 5th—talk to the cancer doctor again

Feb 12th—cardio echo here in Tyler to make sure his thrombus isn't coming back already since being off Coumadin

Feb 20th—pre-op appointments with anesthesiologist/surgeon

Feb 21st—surgery.

Then hanging out in Houston for at least a week.

Then recheck

After recheck

After recheck.

27 January 2008 at 12:50am

Good news (I think) is that the place I've got my car financed through has re-financed it for a lower rate and just a little higher payments and that's allowed us over $2,000 towards our current and upcoming expenses.

It's depressing that I get to start my 5-year loan ALL OVER again a year and a half into it, but I'm grateful that we even had this option.

They also gave us a line of credit for up to $5,000 over the next three years, which should pretty much do it for rechecks, our trip up north for my older son Dave's college graduation, and our vacation this summer.

31 January 2008 17 12:17am

Ward's birthday. Every day together is a gift.

I don't know what horrible things he did in a past life to earn himself such health problems AND *me* as a wife in this life, but I know that *I* must've done something very right my last go-around.

04 February 2008 at 10:17pm

Well, they've changed everything up on us.

Instead of one appointment tomorrow we've got three, so we'll be home LATE tomorrow night, and they've changed his surgery date from the 21st to the 22nd, but we're getting all the pre-ops tomorrow so don't have to come back till the night before surgery.

Ward's still up at the hospital—he started with blood work at 1:15pm and is getting his CAT scan right now—we'll go pick him up in a little bit (I hope).

Because of the different test requirements and limitations, we had to run back to the hotel in between his X-rays and his MRI and have "dinner" at about 3pm.

At least we'll have the really bad storms they are predicting to drive through on the way home.

That'll help keep us awake.

05 February 2008 at 11:25pm

We're home.

The big scary storms moved in a line southeasterly as we moved in
a line northwesterly, and we literally snuck under them going
across Lake Livingston as the sun set.

Really pretty in a creepy, dangerous sort of way.

It rained on us a bit, but that's it. Brownsboro is OK, but I'm
watching the news where they are showing hail damage in Lindale
and Bullard—both less than 30 miles from us.

In Houston, they moved Ward's pre-op appointments to today, so
we got out later than expected—we left Houston at 3:30pm and
stopped for supper (AFTER being clear of the storms).

The blood work, x-rays and CAT scan are what the plastic surgeon
needs before surgery, and the MRI shows STILL NO CANCER
which is very, very, very, very good.

They changed his surgery date to the 22nd, so we'll be going down
the morning of the 21st and will see the anesthesiologist that
afternoon. They anticipate the surgery will take about 7 hours.

I HATE the waiting room.

21 February 2008 at 9:52pm

We're here.

We left the house at 8:30 this morning, got to the hospital at
2:30pm for his 2:45pm appointment, finally SAW the

anesthesiologist at 4:30pm, and now we're headed to bed, to be all rested for our surgery check in time tomorrow at 5:15am.

Oy.

I had another breakdown right here—between the last entry and leaving for surgery.

Just couldn't stand the thought of Ward going under the knife...again.

Ward comforted me, holding me and telling me everything was going to be OK. Then he stopped, kind of chuckled, and said, "Hey. I'm the one being operated on tomorrow—why am I comforting YOU?"

I glared at him through tears and stated, "You are SO selfish—this is so not about you, this is about ME".

I'm a terrible person.

22 February 2008 at 9:00pm

We've been back at the hotel for an hour. We were up at 3:30 this morning and Ward was in surgery from 7:30am-4: 30pm.

I was first allowed to see him at 6pm, but Alec was not. When we left the hospital, he was still in recovery, but they were hoping to move him to ICU by 9pm, where he is to stay for at least 24 hours.

He looks like he's been hit by a truck.

A very big truck.

-He's got the grafted area, which is bigger than before because they had to get "new margins."
-He's got an incision from his chin to just under his ear where they pulled a vein.
-He's got an incision from his armpit to his waist where they took the graft tissue.
-He's got a square "road burn" where they took skin to cover the new graft.

For some reason, his one poor remaining eyelid is bruised, like they couldn't stand leaving any part of him unmarred.

They shaved both sides of his beautiful beard and left a goatee.

I hate goatees.

The doctor said he was stable throughout surgery and did bleed less, but not A LOT less, and that the graft was.... tricky.

He sounded guarded about the prognosis for this one being "the end of this mess."

We are very, very tired and are headed to bed.

23 February 2008 at 11:00am

They called when they moved Ward into ICU from recovery—they didn't get his blood pressure where they wanted it till about 10pm. Then I went directly to sleep and stayed that way till about 7 this morning.

I've talked to his nurse, and to Ward, and we are taking showers (I let Alec sleep in) and then headed to the grocery store for provisions—haven't done that yet.

Then lunch and to the hospital.

Alec won't be able to see Ward, but we did get clearance from the Child Social Worker for him to be in the waiting room in ICU for the 30 minutes I'll be able to visit him. Alec has talked to Ward on the phone twice—once last night, and once this morning.

Then to pick up poor Spooj, who's been at doggy daycare since Thursday evening.

It DOES bite to be the only grownup down here and there are limits on who can go where.

I know that recovery room always looks rough. We've done it before. And that's what's so upsetting—that we keep thinking, "THIS is the last time we have to go through this," and then it starts all over again.

I cannot fathom my husband's bravery and courage, or my son's patience and hope.

I only endeavor to be half the person they are when I grow up.

24 February 2008 at 9:30am

Yesterday afternoon was hard.

I ping ponged every 15 minutes between ICU and the waiting room (meaning washing hands on the way out of ICU, then before going back in again), bouncing from poor Ward, who is still all swollen and puffy and who is still hooked up to all sorts of stuff and who doesn't WANT to be left alone (and has post-anesthetic depression) and poor Alec, who I set up in a corner of the crowded waiting area with his book and a bottle of water and who didn't WANT (understandably) to be left all alone in there.

After the first few go-arounds, both computers in the waiting room were unoccupied, so I let Alec get on Big Phish Games on one, with strict instructions that if an adult got on the other one he was to go immediately back to his corner so there would be one available for another adult.

Then we got to doggy daycare just in time to free Spooj, who was VERY happy to see us.

I've talked to Ward this morning, and he sounds some better. They are talking about getting him moved to a regular room sometime today, but we've learned that the time it takes from talking about it to actually doing it is usually substantial. Hopefully by tonight.

It's supposed to be almost 80 and sunny here today,

And doggy daycare is closed, so we are having breakfast, getting showers and heading up to the hospital before it's too warm to leave Spooj in the car in the parking garage.

Then we'll come back to the hotel, have some lunch and try to find the Dog Park Farouq at doggy daycare told us about.

24 February 2008 at 6:01pm

They moved Ward into a regular room (is it bad when all the nurses on the floor recognize you?) at about 3pm. , and Alec was VERY happy to see his dad, even with all the disturbing drains, stitches, wrappings and various colors he is (Betadine blue, iodine orange, etc). The swelling has gone down some, and they have him sitting up in a chair.

They did take his "on demand" morphine button away from him, which always makes him very sad.

We found the dog park, and even though Spooj was unimpressed with the company (she spent the entire 3 hours sleeping under my bench with her back firmly to the happy playing puppies), Alec found 4 new friends to run rampant with on the very nice playground (for the young human variety). I hope that he'll go to bed early tonight, so I can too. Of course, right now he's running sprints with a little girl whose family is here at the hotel, so who do I think I'M kidding???

I've gotta say, even though there's NO place in this huge city where it's QUIET, the old neighborhoods surrounding the Medical Complex/Rice University are just lovely—all older houses, all different sizes and styles, little front yards and upstairs balconies absolutely PACKED with flowers, herbs and oriental grasses—none of the sterile lawns and cookie cutter houses of suburbia.

25 February 2008 at 12:28pm

When I called Ward's room this morning, a wonderful thing happened.

I didn't hear the painful croaking of the post-surgical, post-breathing-tube patient I've been visiting ever since Friday night.

Ward answered.

In Ward's voice.

Ward's lovely, loved, quiet, calm deep sexy voice.

We've just finished the laundry (Alec had a strange aversion to going out today wearing only his boxer shorts—go figure) and now I'll get my shower, feed the boy lunch and knowledge, but as soon as we are done

we're going to see Daddy.

26 February 2008 at 8:58pm

Well, he's slowly looking better. They took out one of his drains today...three to go.

They are making noises like they are going to release him tomorrow or Thursday, but we have to come back NEXT Wednesday to get the rest of the drains out and start some suture removal.

Whatever.

We're ready to go home...

27 February 2008 at 1:45pm

Apparently they ARE letting him go this afternoon. They've called his scripts to the pharmacy and taken him to the basement beauty shop to get his mane untangled and washed (hopefully he won't look so much like Nick Nolte's mug shot when I go up there).

I'll be taking Spooj AND Alec to doggy daycare and then getting Ward checked out and settled at the hotel.

Alec has been hired (he says his title is Unpaid Intern) by doggy daycare- he walks dogs, hoses out runs, feeds, waters, washes dishes, fetches dogs for clients, helps with lawn work, and generally hangs out. Today the groomer is there, and she has already lined up a few dogs for him to wash...

After his first afternoon there, the owner remarked that since Alec's used to doing chores at home, he knows how to feed, water, make sure gates are closed behind him and read animals' body language—so he's a better hand than most adults they hire and he's welcome anytime.

Although he loves seeing his dad, sitting in the hospital room is mind-killingly boring for ME, I can't imagine how bad it is for Alec. And with all the times we've been to the hospital, he's pretty much played out the video games in the kids' room, so we're grateful that he's got something HE can do that's a real accomplishment while we are here.

27 February 2008 at 10:53pm

Well, our hotel room is once again holding all four of us.

Spooj is asleep at my feet and the boys are watching Smash Lab on Discovery Channel.

Headed home tomorrow.

28 February 2008 at 6:47pm

Home.

Tired.

Later.

05 March 2008 at 8:26pm

Good.

The doctor says good.

We got one of the drains out, and can pull the other one at home in a few days (ick). They took all the sutures out of his neck and side. He finished up his antibiotics and doesn't need any more. They took out the packing in his nose. The graft on his head and the donor site on his leg are healing and we don't have to keep them covered any more, just moisturized.

And bestest of all, he's been cleared for taking normal showers again.

The doctor wants to see him back in two weeks to take out the final drain and make sure everything is progressing nicely.

We drove down yesterday, saw the doctor today, and drove back this afternoon.

I'm tired.
Ward's exhausted.
Spooj is delirious.
Alec is fine.

11 March 2008 at 11:26am

Nuthin' too dramatic to report—that's a GOOD thing.

Ward's back at work almost full time—he gets up at the regular time, but there's still a fair to-do getting him all done and presentable...and he's not rushing, so he gets there about 10ish instead of 9.

The incisions look good. The one on his side is shedding something that looks for all the world like a little bitty snakeskin. His shoulder on that side is really sore—I guess both from the healing and the fact that he's missing a hunk of muscle there now.

His drain on his side is ready to be taken out—I'll do that tomorrow (the measurable drainage has to be below 30cc in a 24 hour period for 3 consecutive days, and today is the 3rd day for that)(and no, I don't remember anything in the marriage vows that say "I promise to strip, drain, measure the fluids and re-set body cavity drains," but there it is...), but the one on his head has been draining A LOT more. Since surgery, it hadn't had more than 4cc's per 24 hours. In the last two days, it's been *18 and 30* cc's respectively.

The swelling below the graft was huge and has now gone down visibly, so hopefully that's what it is. Interestingly, this happened right after his first good sneeze (which he's supposed to avoid).

It would be bad if that made a new hole behind the graft (but we don't think it did since the drain is still holding suction), but too funny if it blew out whatever needed to get out of the way so his face can return to normal size.

15 March 2008 at 10:30pm

He's started to seep stuff right THROUGH the graft—looks like tears.... or drool.... something clear and watery, sweating out through the pores.

Nothing in the drain. Just this weird seepage. And only when he chews. Which was very attractive at Schlotzky's today. It was actually dripping onto his shirt.

Called the doctor and they said that if he's not running fever, and it's not coming from the incision, and it's not bloody or otherwise yakky, that it's probably something from his still swollen cheek/jaw trying to get out, but if it's still doing it tomorrow they'll call in some preventive antibiotics and unless the whole shebang literally blows off, they'll see us as scheduled on Wednesday morning.

We are so frustrated, discouraged, exhausted, and otherwise fed up we can hardly stand it.

16 March 2008 at 4:01pm

Hmmm..... received this info from a friend:

POSSIBLE COMPLICATIONS

Skin grafting carries risks and potential complications that vary based on the type of wound being treated and the location of the skin graft on the body. Complications may include:

-Graft failure;
-Rejection of the skin graft;
-Infections at donor or recipient sites;
-Blood buildup underneath the graft;

-Fluid weeping from graft sites;
-Autograft donor sites oozing fluid and blood as they heal
-Scarring;
-Hyperpigmentation, or the presence of color;
-Blood clots;
-Skin redness surrounding the graft site;
-Pain; and
-Re-ulceration, or the development of new ulcers on the same limb.

He's had 10 out of 12 of those.

So far.

17 March 2008 at 10:15pm

I emailed some photos to the doctor this morning, along with an update, so he's got a 'heads-up' for Wednesday, and he emailed back that he wants blood work and a CAT scan...BEFORE the appointment.

So instead of planning on being gone 24 hours, we have to assume we may be delayed through the weekend (or beyond...).

Therefore, I had to take the puppy to be boarded, get to the feed store, set up work where they need to be, and get Ward's scripts filled for that amount of time.

And instead of a leisurely morning packing and leaving out after lunch, we'll be up early and gone by 9am to make it to the hospital before 2pm.

Luckily, it's gonna be thunder storming all the way down there to help keep me awake.

19 March 2008 at 7:10pm

Home. We're home.

They said the graft looks ok—a little sinusitis accounting for the pussy chunkiness, but nothing terrible. They put him on 10 days worth of antibiotics.

His blood work came back all right, so it's nothing systemic.

The swelling in his cheek was a cyst—maybe a blocked salivary gland from all the messing about they've done in there. They drained over 30cc's from it and his face looks better.

It MIGHT come back up, in which case we'll have to go back to have it drained again—the surgeon said he doesn't want anyone else poking around so close to the graft—but it should eventually dry up on it's own and stop it.

Otherwise the doctor does NOT want to see us till June. (And he sounded a little threatening...)

Mar 28 2008, 10:55 PM

Ward got fired today.

It's ok.

He's felt stuck there because of his age/condition/need for insurance, but he hated it for a good 5 of the 8 years he was there.

They did give him severance and 2 months paid insurance, so we'll have time for unemployment/COBRA to kick in (I may put him on MY work insurance, may be cheaper than COBRA).

And the funny thing (?) is that he applied for disability last week. They told him he needed to keep his income below a certain level and we were going to have a problem...

He doesn't have another doctor's appointment till June, but he DOES need to see about physical therapy—his side is messed up from missing a muscle there for the donor tissue, and his face is still paralyzed from surgery.

AND Alec has a tournament in Alabama that we wanted him to be able to compete in in April AND we have David's college graduation in May in Minnesota AND Ward really needs some time to just HEAL and he wasn't sure how to be able to take all this extra time off.

His boss asked him if there was anything he could do to help him (they are getting rid of the warehouse part of the business and just drop-shipping everything- so no need for an Inventory Manager anymore...) and Ward just looked at him and said, "I think you just did".

He already looks and sounds 10 years younger.

Says he feels like he's got his whole life ahead of him.

Says he's scared outta his pants.

So, except for a few pesky details (what's a few more???), it's OK.

24 April 2008 at 9:36am

A good thing.

A very good thing.

We found out yesterday that he's been approved for Social Security Disability effective back to November of '07.

We are still in shock—we just applied for SSD four weeks ago and had heard that it would take at least 2 go arounds, over a year, and a good lawyer to get approved.

We were both positive that there must be a catch. It must be a clerical error.

The only things that happen quickly and easily for us are bad things, and if a good thing DOES happen, it's usually followed by a bad thing of equal or greater value.

We talked to the caseworker and it's not an error. It's real and for true.

And last night it finally occurred to me: maybe THIS good thing has been pre-paid by what we've already been through...

And we feel much better.

10 June 2008 at 12:03am

Tomorrow we head back to Houston for quarterly appointments, scans, and blood work.

We'll be gone till late Friday.

If they tell us "something" is back and they have to mess up this finally perfectly healed graft, I'm gonna have to hurt somebody.

Really.

11 June 2008 at 9:35pm

First appointment. Plastic surgeon says the graft looks good and he
doesn't want to see us again till our next appointment with the
cancer doctor.

Tomorrow are the scans, and Friday (the 13th) is the scary
appointment with the cancer doctor.

Although I would *hope* that the graft would look sketchy (like
before) if there were any aberrant activity going on under there...

Tonight we splurged at Barnes and Noble and I bought TWO
books (one on cabins and another on rock work) that are the first
books I've bought EVER that weren't used from Amazon or on the
deep discount shelves. Looking and planning for our new place is
what's kept me from going stark raving mad this last year. And my
not being stark raving mad is very helpful for everyone's safety and
sanity.

Then we went to a tiny little Sicilian family restaurant, another
splurge—more than we've EVER spent on one meal, but we
brought home enough for tomorrow night's dinner AND it was
Absolutely. Completely. Divine.

The restaurant is built right into the family home, and we were
serenaded by the patriarch, who quietly sits in a corner with a glass
of wine and sings beautiful songs in Italian and plays his guitar.
I'm half Sicilian and grew up spending summers in the kitchen of a
Sicilian dinner club in central Wisconsin, so this was very, very
soothing. We all had wonderful food we don't normally enjoy, and
the boys got a little peek into my past, as I could sing snippets here
and there and hum along with a lot of the songs.

12 June 2008 at 8:54pm

We went to Geopalooza at the Museum of Natural Science this morning. It was COOL—geodes taller than Alec, HUGE fossils (even some pterodactyls), a section where the kids could "pan" for gemstones. Alec snagged some good-sized amethysts and hematites, and several smaller bits of garnet, tiger's eye, and agate.

Then he got to choose a geode to have cracked open. He stood at the bin and felt each one, "listening" to see if it seemed right, then took the one that "spoke" to him up to the cutter. They had the sample ones there with a few little crystals—you were guaranteed one with "something" inside, but every time I've done it in the past the "something" has been a few lumps of grey stuff—nothing to write home about.

They cracked it open.

It's gorgeous.

Filled completely with fully formed, multi-faceted lavender crystals.

Then we dropped Alec off to work at doggy daycare and we went on to the hospital for Ward's scans.

Tomorrow is THE appointment...

I think we'll all sleep with a lavender crystal under our pillows.

13 June 2008 at 8:46pm

Home.

We're home.

The radiologist who reads all Dr. Hanna's stuff is out this week, but Dr. Hanna and three of his colleagues looked at the MRI and all said

LOOKS CLEAR.

And they don't want to see us again for 4 months.

AND there were two new litters of baby guinea pigs born while I was gone—ALL Merinos—a rare breed that only a handful of people in the US are working on, and I'm one of them.

AND there were 19 baby chicks waiting in the incubator for me when I got home.

Ok, I'm gonna go feed critters and boys now.

Oct 29 2008, 11:15 AM

So. It's been 4 months...

Once again we packed the car, but this time we headed *northeast* for the National Taekwondo tournament in Chattanooga, where Alec solidly earned a bronze medal in Traditional Form and a GOLD medal in Freestyle Form.

Chattanooga put us within cat-swingin' distance of Princess Bootcamp Headquarters—a get-together from an online forum I'm involved with, soooooo... After a wonderful visit with people I feel closer to than most of my 'normal' family we turned the car towards Houston.

The plastic surgeon said that after almost two long years and two attempts, the graft we now have is "a keeper," and unless something goes wrong underneath it, he doesn't want to see us again.... ever.

Ward got his MRI, but the cancer doctor had gotten called out of town, so we just got the results this morning—

Results of last week's MRI show

NOTHING OF NOTE IN WARD'S HEAD.

NO recurrence of tumor activity.

They'll schedule an appointment for another MRI 4-6 months out, but until then...

...We're good to go.

2009

24 April 2009 at 11:53pm

Ward—ups and downs, mentally and physically. Still better than
when he was working, though. They've cut him to every 6 months
instead of every 3 months for scans, which is wonderful and scary
both. He's got scans next week and we're all a little twitchy about
that. If "something" shows up, I don't know what we'll do—we had
to drop his insurance in March when they raised the premium so
high there was no way to afford it. He's insurance-free till
November when Medicare kicks in. 'Course, that's the least of it—I
don't know how our family could deal with yet another go-around
with the Big C. Ward's been so brave and been through so much—
there's no one on Earth I admire more, or love more fiercely.

Alec is great. Now a first degree level two black belt AND
instructor, he got his World Champion chevron in Freestyle form.
Currently on spring break—he'll start his final quarter of 4th grade
home school next week. I gave myself a promotion to Principal
and hired a teacher for him—his dad. It's working terrific. They are
a great team. He inherited his dad's bravery and brains, along with
that quirky dry sense of humor—what a fabulous kid!

20 May 2009 at 9:59pm

Ya.

So two weeks ago they did a routine cancer scan and it was ALL
CLEAR. Cancer doctor said, "Go home and have a wonderful
summer. See you in November."

Yesterday, the graft—the beautiful 15-month-old, perfectly healed
graft, sprung a hole. One of the interior staples worked its way to
the surface and, on the entire graft, it chose to make a hole
right
where
it's failed before.

Every time.

Three surgery's worth.

There's no tissue there—it's right on what's left of his brow bone.

There's whistling from the hole to the sinus.

We're waiting for the doctor to call/e-mail us back, but I'm 99.5%
sure we're headed back to Houston in the next week.

Good thing he still has insurance, or I'd be REALLY stressed.

Oh.

No wait.

He doesn't.

22 May 2009 at 11:14pm

The staple fell out, but the hole is bigger and rimmed with red.
He's running a low-grade fever and his blood sugar has spiked to
300—all signs of infection. That whole side of his head hurts really

badly—he said, "My head kind of hurts," which means, if it were me, I'd be rolling in agony. The man never complains of pain.

The soonest the doctor can see him is Wednesday morning (thank you, Holiday Weekend), but he called in antibiotics, which Ward started taking today. Until then he's to keep it clean and do nothing that would get it dirty or sweaty or cause more damage, like lifting and straining.

Ya. This IS the weekend we are supposed to finish mulching the garden and set up the watering system...

Luckily I have two other helpers and Ward can supervise—although he's really feeling depressed because he was just now starting to be up for physical labor.

In addition to Alec, we now have Joe, who we met in Georgia at the Princess Bootcamp and whom we've now adopted. Life's funny that way.

So—back to Houston Tuesday afternoon and our appointment Wednesday morning.
I just want him better. I just want to be able to stop worrying. He's a good man—nay, the BEST man—on Earth. Kind, funny, sexy, smart, and loving,

and seven years of this crap is

Just. Too. Much.

26 May 2009 at 9:05am

I need to run about a million errands including putting in some time at work, but hope to load the troops and be outta here by 3pm (insert hysterical laughter).

We're taking Spooj with us—she started limping something fierce and I can't have Joe (with his bad knee—HIS surgery is NEXT month) carrying her up and down the stairs. So I've got her on low dose aspirin, which seems to help.

I figured out her age. She's at least 16.

Will. Not. Think. About. That.

Joe's got instructions on feeding the two-week-old chicks in their nursery in the henhouse and turning the eggs in the incubator. And my TURKEYS are supposed to come tomorrow morning,

I carefully timed all this poultry activity so I'd BE HERE for it...

Can't say Ward's head hurts any less, but I've been tossing him one of my Special Migraine Big Pink Pills every night—he spends a few hours laughing at stupid stuff on the internet, so I think they're helping some.

He's also been bleeding off and on without warning—both from the graft and his nose, on accounta they're connected by the hole—which is disturbing in several different ways...

27 May 2009 at 7:02pm

Home. We're home.

The doctor walked in and said "Mr. Dixon, you have a hole in your head. That'll be $200."

No. Not really.

It was more like $250.

They looked. They examined. They said:

-The hole itself, from the graft out through his nose, won't kill him.
-It may close on its own, but probably not. The bigger likelihood is
that *if* it heals, it'll heal open—even so far as to grow "outside"
skin on the inside.
-The graft is not in danger, but he needs to be careful with it so it
doesn't get too dirty or open bigger.
-If he gets more infections, they'll try to treat with more antibiotics
till November.
-Come November (when he starts getting Medicare), they'll
probably send him to the prosthetics department and they can
fashion a plug for the hole so it won't be open anymore.
-He's not too worried about an abscess forming, since it's open on
both ends and gravity will keep the bottom end from closing before
the top end.

The doctor said, "I'll go look at the scans, but it seems pretty
straightforward and I don't expect to see anything—come back in
November".

5 minutes later he was back.

There's another air pocket behind the graft—not a problem NOW,
but we need to be REALLY, REALLY CAREFUL that the hole
doesn't get bigger. If it does, we'll have to plug it NOW or risk
losing the graft.

So. Not. Going. There.

We at least know now exactly what we're dealing with, how to care
for it, and what to watch for.

The antibiotics he's on right now are wreaking havoc on Ward's
tummy and he (*and I*) haven't slept more than two hours at a
stretch since this started a week ago. Ward slept all the way home,
and I'm headed that way right after dinner, I think (I hope).

Kinda puts the kibosh on heavy-duty gardening and building projects, but we'll make do.

30 July 2009 at 11:01am

ARRRRGGGHHHHH!!!!!!

My last post here was May 27th. Things were looking up.

The antibiotics worked—the infection went away and Ward started putting one of those little round band-aids over the hole to keep the air from actually flowing through it (air flow = making the hole bigger by breathing/sneezing/snoring etc).

We took our trip to Montana and all parts in between, which was grand. (Yes, even though we went up there to be with Joe during his surgery—bankrolled in large part by Joe—as soon as we knew he was in the clear, we abandoned him like yesterday's newspaper and went vacationing. Cuz that's just how we roll...)

During the trip, the hole actually CLOSED ITSELF UP. Looked great—not a scab, but actual healed lovely skin.

Three days ago the hole blew open again.

YESTERDAY he told me about it.

(He tends to fall asleep with his glasses on, since he reads in bed and his patch is attached to his glasses, so I didn't see it).

I said, "And exactly WHEN were you going to tell me about this???"

He sheepishly said, "Ummm...now?"

Remember when your toddlers would cover their OWN eyes and say, "You can't see me?" That's my darling beloved dear husband's attitude. If he doesn't TELL me something's wrong, it's not.

It's bigger. Before, it was about 1/2 inch in diameter. Now it's 1/2 inch high but an inch long—running along the suture line, oozing from inside, red angry skin around it.

He's back on antibiotics, and back to being extra very careful about dirt/lifting/etc.

We're looking at huge changes at work, Joe's up in Montana facing HIS post-surgical stuff, we've got people coming to look at our house NEXT FRIDAY and it's a horror,
we've just got the garden replanted over yonder and THAT needs tending, IF the house sells we'll be MOVING INTO A STRUCTURE THAT'S NOT EVEN THERE YET, but HEY!

I'm fine. Really.

10 August 2009 at 10:57pm

Appointment schedule-

Monday 8am plastic surgeon,

12:30 lab work,

3pm CT scan

Tuesday 8am cancer doctor

Good thing we don't have to pay up front for it.

Oh.

No.

Wait.

17 August 2009 at 8:39pm

Today's anecdote:

I spent literally hours last week arranging our visit to MDAnderson today and tomorrow to assure no more emotional stress on my family than necessary.

Since we are pre-pay right now, I wanted to know the exact amount I needed to bring with us.

Since LAST time, when I paid by money order in the morning, it still wasn't posted in the afternoon and they almost told us we couldn't have the scan we'd just forked over $2,000+ dollars for till I called and raised Cain about it, I arranged to deliver the money straight to the business office lady this time—in cash.

The business office lady told me the exact amount we'd need for scan, blood work, swabs, and office visits for two doctors. We repeated that number back to each other at least three times, and I brought about $50 extra.

The business office lady told me that since our first doctor's appointment was at 8am and she doesn't get there till 9am, we should go to the doctor's, then to her to pay, then proceed to the other stuff.

We got to the doctor's appointment at 7:45am and were told we couldn't see him—there was a lock on the account because we're pre-pay. We were also told that the actual amount needed was over $300 MORE than what I was quoted.

We got informed of all of this in the middle of the waiting room, surrounded by other patients and staff.

I asked, calmly, if there wasn't somewhere ELSE we could discuss this matter.

So I left a child with anxiety issues and a husband who already feels like he's ruined us financially AND who's on narcotic pain medication in the waiting room and proceeded to politely but firmly work my way through that lady, her supervisor, the supervisor at the business office, and the gal I'd been talking to.

Over an hour. Took over an hour.

And a goodly part of that was explaining that no I COULDN'T leave my husband and child to see the doctor by themselves and go directly to pay—I HAVE to be with them. Ward's on narcotics and fuzzy and Alec's nine. *I* need to be able to talk to the doctor and hear what he says in person.

That I had brought exactly what I had been told to bring and was doing things in exactly the order I'd been told to do them and I was very sorry for their confusion but that I expected them to uphold their end of what they had told me to do, and that YES we would be seeing the doctor and that NO I didn't need to find an extra $300 right that minute.

In the end, the doctor saw us, and the amount I brought was fine, and we were able to proceed with the rest of the tests and appointments.

From the plastic surgeon's exam, we learned that his concerns include keeping the infections from coming back (Ward has what amounts to an extra sinus with that hole behind his graft) and to keep him from hurting too much while not getting addicted to narcotics. His MAIN concern, because of the bleeding and the pain, is that the tumors are back—and they have nowhere to go but into his brain.

Of course the business office lady was quick to point out that if we need to go to surgery we'd need to find a whole MESS of money before they'd to that.

Thanks.

Because we'd nevera thought of THAT. It's never in our every thought, waking or sleeping, that IF it comes back and IF it's operable that we need hundreds of thousands of dollars or he'll just have to die.

18 August 2009 at 6:41pm

We're home.

No Cancer

That's mainly what I wanted to hear. No Cancer.

Those words that make me smile when the doctor walks into the room and says, "Dixons—I've reviewed the scans and find nothing going on in Ward's head."
They swabbed the hole, and are having him irrigate it every day. He still has directives to not get dirt in it OR breathe dirt or spores or dust or hair or anything else we waller in unless he wears a mask, since contaminants can enter that "extra sinus" from both the hole AND that nostril.

They want to see us in four months for more scans and to figure a game plan on fixing said hole. Till then, we keep it clean and treat infection and pain as they occur.

We love all our friends from around the world for rallying round and sending emails and letters to MDAnderson about their payment policies. The scary thing is that our case isn't even BAD. Our loved one isn't dying or dead, we aren't bankrupt or homeless. So many people have had a much tougher go—not only there, but also at hospitals all over the country—needing TENS of thousands of dollars up front.

I'm thinking that people like us, like me, are the ones who will be able to change that, though—the others are just too beaten down by worry or give up when their loved one dies.

19 August 2009 at 4:59pm

Ha.

So I called Patient Advocacy as requested, asked for "our" assigned person by name as requested, and got her voicemail.

But patient service is their main goal, and my call is VERY important to them.

20 August 2009 at 12:20am

Interesting....

On the MDAnderson website, their Code of Ethics #10:

"Cancer therapy, prevention, education, and research are costly endeavors demanding conscientious stewardship; however, financial considerations should not dictate the quality of care offered to each patient."

Wow.

20 August 2009 at 8:55pm

Hahahaha. Ms. H****** has not returned my calls, even though I identified myself and gave the details over the phone to her answering machine.

The message said, "If you are calling after 4pm (I was), your call will be returned before noon the following business day". It's now 8pm of the next day and I carry my phone with me.

Let me be very, very clear—we've always been 150% happy with the staff at MDA. The doctors are the greatest, and the nursing staff is amazing.

Even the business office personnel are just saying what they are being told from above.

What needs addressed is the now-so-obvious fact that the administration has gone beyond the original intent of the hospital and their very own Code of Ethics.

The waste is phenomenal—literally tens of thousands of square feet just for walking through or lounging, acres of waiting rooms and areas that are never used. I've walked the whole dang thing at all hours of the day and night.

All we can think of is that it's there for show, to "prove" what a World Class Facility they have. We'd be far more impressed with a compact facility that keeps its eye on the real purpose—to provide care for all patients with respect and compassion, and without regard for ability to pay.

I don't have a problem with new labs, surgical suites, or equipment and places to put them.

I have a problem with acres of NOTHING all in public areas— hundreds (maybe thousands?) of sofas and palm trees as far as the eye can see.

And everywhere you turn is some huge sign, display, or exhibit that rivals any museum, showing their history, goals, and most of all accomplishments—stating with no bones about it that they NEED more money or their fight against cancer will be lost.

Interestingly, I've never seen the Code of Ethics posted anywhere except buried in the website.

25 August 2009 at 9:23am

An update:

I called H****** at askMDA as requested Monday morning. I asked for her by name and was told "she's unavailable, but let me take your number." And she did call back. She figured out who our *actual* Patient Advocate is in the Head and Neck Center and left *her* a message to call me.

T*******, our Patient Advocate, called me that afternoon, and she and I had a nice little chat for about an hour.

She's filing a formal complaint, and is checking into what may be available for us as far as financial help. I relayed to her that our disappointment in the Best Cancer Hospital in the World is NOT and never has been with the doctors or nurses, or even (mostly) the other staff members.

But considering their very publicly stated pride in making sure every patient is treated as an individual and given specially drawn up treatment plans, it's disappointing that when we, as established patients, presented with a medical problem related to (not caused by—we are not placing blame for the hole in his head, we just want it fixed) their treatment, and that we happen to be in between insurance coverage, I was asked how much our annual income is and that was the only and final determinant for financial aid.

Denied.

Pre-pay at time of service.

Have a nice day.

I pointed out that even though our income has not changed substantially since we started this cancer dance seven years ago— my one raise in pay being balanced by his job loss and going on disability—our RESOURCES are wildly different:

Savings? Gone.
Retirement accounts? Gone.
Paid-for house? Equitied out THREE times.
Credit card? Maxed to the hilt with medical expenses.
Credit score due to outstanding medical bills (which exceed $100,000 even though we HAD insurance for all but the last 6 months)? Dismal.

I explained that our pre-pay status was not a problem for our normally scheduled scan in May—we knew about it, understood the non-emergency (but important to keep up with all the same) nature of that visit, and saved up for it. As the manager of an animal emergency clinic, I understand that there are expenses in running a medical facility.

But:

That MDAnderson is a TEACHING hospital, in a State University system, and receives federal funding to operate. That we are Texas residents, who are supposed to receive preferred status care (it being a TEXAS university hospital and all...),

And that at this point in time, with National Health Care so prominent in the news, this is not even JUST about my family— what we're going through isn't even BAD compared to a lot of folks who go literally bankrupt and still lose their loved one.

How can they tell people "pay or die?"

Here's what she said, and what she's checking into:

They shouldn't.

They CAN, in certain instances, bump cases further up than the business office, and apply for Medical Override, which would waive charges for a certain procedure or amount of time.

In our case, where though the problem did not present during the normal post-surgical time frame, the integrity of the graft has always been the bugaboo—and this SHOULD have been bumped up for review since, by law, once they start treatment for something, they cannot refuse to finish. Period.

What she's looking into will be getting us Medical Override till he goes on Medicare in November—taking the 'how will we pay for it?' stress off of my family.

Which is huge.

Just the knowledge that we CAN go down there if we need to without scrambling, neglecting other bills, or borrowing from already depleted friends and family may very well be enough to allow Ward to relax, and heal on his own.

26 August at 10:54pm

Well, the nurse called today. They've finished growing Ward's Garden O' Germs and have found that he's got another staph infection.

Since the Augmentin didn't touch it this go around, they've put him on two week's worth of Bactrim.

(Off to buy up cases of yogurt...)

05 September 2009 at 4:06pm

So.

I gave our Advocate the week to make our lives better.

(Insert shaking head and polite chuckling.)

Back when all this mess started, we told the business office that we had insurance—good insurance—but that we had no resources to throw at what would remain of our bill(s) till

a) Our house sold or
b) We were through this mess, and wouldn't have all those pesky peripherals to worry about—lodging, gas, food, travel and existing expenses—for going down yonder, and could start making monthly payments on the balance due.

They were fine with that.

But apparently that's what's put the lock on our account—that we have an outstanding balance with MDA from when we had insurance.

Never mind that we've thrown well over $5,000 in cash at them for our scans in May and the ones just recently. That "doesn't show good faith."

I was told that if I made payment arrangements to put a minimum amount on the existing balance, starting NOW, that would take the lock off of our account.

Whatever.

Our advocate told me to call the billing office, since the business office doesn't make payment arrangements.

The billing office told me to call the business office, since the billing office doesn't place the locks on accounts.

I finally worked my way through to the billing office person in charge of business office accounts. (And yes, I did need a migraine pill by that time.)

We've made arrangements for monthly payments—made the first one over the phone even.

Now I'll call back to the business office on Tuesday to see if the lock's been lifted.

Oh.

And the "medical over-ride?"

IF they unlock the account, it'll go into effect, but it's not "Here—let us treat you for free if you need our services from now thru October," it's more of a "You can come in to be treated if you need our services and we'll be happy to tack the full amount onto the bottom of your existing bill."

Thanks.

Ward's hole looks better, but he's really painful again, not hungry at all, and the antibiotics are kicking his digestive tract's butt.

He sleeps most of the time and looks very thin to me.

06 September 2009 at 10:04am

Yanno, we've been really more than 100% happy with the MEDICAL care we've gotten at MDA, even with the usual "going through channels" irritations that sometimes crop up. The issues have only been with the financial end of it.

And I'm making sure Ward gets yogurt at least once a day (wish I were milking now and had goat milk yogurt, but we are using the stuff with added probiotics) and basically, whenever he expresses a desire for ANY food, I make sure he gets it.

I know he hurts because of the infection and his tummy's upset because of the antibiotics and he's sleeping because of the narcotics for the pain, but he's so tired of this whole particular circle that he's also really, really crabby, and that's SO understandable, but SO not like him, which affects Alec, who worries so much and gets his feelers hurt so much, cuz that's his DAD who is the GOOD, PATIENT parent, and if DAD'S crabby, all he's left with is
Mean
Old
Mom

06 September 2009 at 6:53pm

We're getting Alec ready for starting his 5th year of home school tomorrow.

Ward wanted to know why I box up EVERYTHING Alec does—workbooks, spelling tests, math problems, science experiments, everything.

I told him it's so when/if CPS comes calling after getting the report that there's a filthy little boy running wild in nothing but boxer shorts, communing with turkeys and perching in trees, we can prove we're really schooling him in between adventures and inventing weapons of rusty destruction from rocks and baling wire.

I AM wore down. I think, from my symptoms, that the endometriosis they scraped out when they did 3 other major surgeries (one being a total hysterectomy) is back.

So I commanded Ward to come keep my back and tummy warm and we both took a two-hour nap.

...Which sounds lovely, except I'm the world's worst napper. I wake up all crabby. So now the boys, dogs, and even the cat from Hell are avoiding me like I'm a rattler with rabies.

09 September 2009 at 4:10pm

In OUR mail today, addressed to Ward:

(It's kinda long, but I wanted to share the whole wonderment with ya'll.)

(Imagine it on ecru MDAnderson letterhead)

Dear Mr. Dixon,

You and MDAnderson are on the threshold!

Yes, that is a bold statement. But it is true.

By making a gift to the MDAnderson Annual Fund, you will stand shoulder to shoulder with our scientists and physicians, who are on the threshold of a transformation in cancer research and care.

You can play a key role in helping to bring the promise of personalized cancer care to your neighbors in the Brownsboro area and all across the nation.

Your support will help us capitalize on recent discoveries in genetics and molecular biology. We are making significant strides in understanding how normal cells become cancerous.

These discoveries are making one-size fits all cancer treatments obsolete. Instead, our goal is to focus on the genetic and molecular blueprints that make each individual cancer- and each individual patient- unique.

The transformational change will take research and resources. *That is why I hope you will help us kick off the 2009-2010 Annual Fund by sending a gift of $20, $50, $75 or more to our Fall Appeal today.*

Your gift is important and deeply appreciated, especially in the current economic climate. If it is at all possible, I hope you will consider making a gift of $100. If you do, you will be recognized as an Anderson Annual Fund Partner at the Century Club level, and you will receive a personalized Certificate of Appreciation.

Whatever the size of your gift, you will be part of medical history. Your support will help us achieve a new level of sophistication in research, bringing together teams of specialists in fields such as immunology, proton therapy, biomedical imaging, and experimental therapeutics.

The collaborative way we organize and manage our pioneering research and patient care programs is part of our vision to transform cancer care.

No other cancer center is incorporating such a transformational method of moving scientific findings to the clinic so quickly.

These scientific discoveries emerge from many interlocking ideas generated by a variety of disciplines and are nurtured by the commitment of friends like you.

You are part of our success in Making Cancer History and I look forward to your support. Thank you again.

Sincerely,
John Mendelsohn MD
President

11 September 2009 at 3:25pm

I'm happy to report that since Ward's finished his antibiotics (he took the last one Tuesday night), his appetite is back and he's grazing up a storm.

22 September 2009 at 10:42pm

So this morning we sat down and figured out a plan.

Our finances have been re-arranged, and we'll be able to siphon several hundred dollars a month towards the new place. Once we have the barn and fences up and a shallow well dug, we can get a little unfinished cabin over there and get moved. If this place hasn't sold by then, we'll rent it out.

In the meanwhile, we'll be really getting rid of a lot of stuff and storing the things we want to keep but that won't fit into the 14 X 30 cabin, making this house more "showable."

It's a plan.

It makes sense.

It would have us moved over yonder in about six months.

One hour later, Ward took his shower and discovered that.

His graft has a new hole in it.

A NEW hole. Not the OLD hole, which is still there.

His OLD hole is at the top of the graft in the upper corner by his nose bone.
His NEW hole is at the top of the graft in the outer corner.
Both are right on the incision line.

We have *39* days till he's on Medicare. Thirty Nine.

Tomorrow, I'll call his doctor and send them a photo. I'll keep sending them photos as things progress (deteriorate?). IF he gets infected, they should be able to prescribe another round of antibiotics.

MY goal is now to keep him held together (literally) till November 1st, when I'm assuming we'll be looking at

A whole

New

Graft.

That's what we get for making plans...

15 October 2009 at 11:33pm

Nov. 3rd, 8am: Cardiologist for stress test/echo and consult re: surgical readiness

Nov. 3rd, 4pm: Drive to Houston

Nov. 4th: Consult with plastic surgeon at MDA to decide best course of action to eradicate holes in Ward's head

Nov. 24th: Surgery date (with pre-ops the day before IF they decide surgery is the way to go with this).

I have hives.

Itchy itchy itchy...

04 November 2009 at 11:44pm

So we went to the cardiologist yesterday, just to be sure before talking to the MDAnderson doctor about how we're going to fix the big honkin' holes in Ward's head that his heart is behaving and fit for another nine hour surgery.

The cardiologist did a chemical stress test, and an echocardiogram, and showed us the full color, full motion video of Ward's heart pumping like a champ.

In spite of the big ol' CLOT that's re-formed on that darn weak spot left by his heart attack all those years ago and that makes a showing every year or so and has to be blasted with a hefty dose of rat poison.

In light of this, the MDAnderson doctor said "Hmmm....lets get rid of the clot. In the meantime, try not to get an infection, and we'll keep our fingers crossed that when they put you on blood thinners it doesn't make the holes bleed TOO much worse than they are now."

Muy helpful.

The main issue right now, besides the clot in his heart, is the pain Ward's been having—sharp burning pains from behind his eye socket down through his teeth on that side, and what feels like tearing around the holes.

They've been giving him Hydrocodone/apap for that since September, and need to get him off of it—not only is the codeine a bad thing to be taking every day (being a NARCOTIC and all...), but he's been ingesting over 3,000mg of Tylenol daily, which is most likely frying his liver.

So they gave him a different prescription with more codeine and less Tylenol till he can see the pain management doctor on Tuesday. (Yes. Tuesday. So we'll be going back down there Monday night). The pain management doctor will most likely do a scan to pinpoint where the affected nerves are and do a nerve block on them—it has to be very precise or Ward'll feel like he's just come from the dentist (with the accompanying lovely drooling) all the time.

So. The plan is:

- Call the cardiologist tomorrow and tell him BLAST THE CLOT, which will take at least a month.

- See the pain doctor next week to make my honey feel better without the aid of narcotics.
- Go to regularly scheduled cancer scan in December
- Once the clot's gone, go back and re-assess our surgery options—they've tentatively scheduled an appointment for that the first week of February.

Here we go again...

18 December 2009 at 8:47pm

I've been remiss with the updates, and for that I apologize. It's been a stressful month or so.

Not long after Ward started the Coumadin again, I noticed he was getting thin (he had been trying to lose a little weight, and was succeeding, but this was coming off WAY too fast. He was eating MORE and looking like a refugee—his pants and wedding ring were falling off).

And that he was sleeping ALL the time, and increasingly difficult to wake.

Now, he WAS starting the Neurontin, which they'd told us would make him really drowsy till his body adjusted to it.

But he just looked really, really bad.

I checked his Codeine/Tylenol supply and it was way too low compared to where it should have been. I asked him about that (he's been taking it at maximum dose since AUGUST, and they reduced the Tylenol amount to avoid liver damage). The Neurontin is supposed to REPLACE the C/T once he works the dosage up, but they gave him a new script for the C/T "for occasional use as needed."

He was still taking what he thought was the maximum dose. He THOUGHT the bottle said "1 or 2 every 4 hours, as needed," or 12 pills a day. What the bottle ACTUALLY said was "1 or 2 four times a day, as needed"—so a maximum of 8 pills. He was overdosing himself on Tylenol by 1,300mg per DAY.

Let's put this in perspective. The safe adult dose of Tylenol is 2,000mg per day for a maximum of 14 days. He'd already been taking 2,600mg per day since AUGUST. And for the 13 days since getting his last script filled, had been taking 3,300mg per day.

Wait.

It gets better.

In my research, I also found that the only thing worse than chronically overdosing yourself on Tylenol is if you mix the Tylenol with

Coumadin.

I freaked.

He freaked.

We got him off of the Codeine/Tylenol (gradually, since codeine is, yanno, an OPIATE).

His doctors did blood work to assess his liver values immediately after this discovery, and the values that have to do with "toxicity—poisoning of the liver" were elevated. His doctors had us STOP the Coumadin till he was weaned off of the C/T.

I weighed him and he weighed 173 pounds. He's 6'2" and SHOULD weigh no less than 185.

He was scheduled for "routine" scans yesterday, and they added liver value blood work to be repeated and an additional scan of his liver. So we've been in Houston the last three days for blood work, CAT and PET scans, and doctor appointments.

The pain doctor changed up his meds to something withOUT Tylenol and doubled the Neurontin, which should almost completely handle the pain issue.

The cancer doctor said that "we" (rolls eyeballs) caught the chronic overdose of Tylenol in time, and since his mean wife took the happy pills away from him, his liver values have already improved 30 points (still 20 away from high normal). There's no permanent liver damage, he's gained back *eight* pounds, and that's all good.

(He also said, "Your wife is brilliant for catching that and acting so quickly " I think I want that embroidered on a pillow or something).

And

He's CANCER FREE from the tip of his pointy little head to his hairy little toes!

19 December 2009 at 2:10pm

Three fun facts I did not know until recently-

-The codeine/Tylenol combo is the THIRD most prescribed medication in the US. Not PAIN medication--ANY medication.

-Worried about health implications of the above mix ('cuz, yanno CODEINE is a "bad drug"), doctors did a study. Three groups of people were dosed—one control group with sugar pills, one group with codeine only, and one group with Tylenol only. The doctors were amazed that the "codeine only" group suffered no adverse effects (after the initial withdrawal "discomfort" from an

OPIATE). The long-term, and sometimes deadly, liver damage was caused 150% by...the Tylenol. One doctor went so far as to say "Codeine/Ibuprofen (Motrin) is an excellent pain killer. Codeine/Tylenol should NEVER be prescribed to anyone, in any form, at any time."

-Of all the many pills someone trying to kill themselves can take, the ones who swallow a big ol' handful of over the counter Tylenol are MOST likely to succeed.

That's what I love about life. There's always something new and exciting to learn.

2010

10 March 2010 at 1:06am

I haven't been on here a lot lately. On top of general busy-ness, Ward's been to the ER twice now in three weeks (the first time he ended up being admitted), and it's looking like we're headed that way again here in a little bit.

He was admitted the night before Alec's birthday. We spent the night at the hospital, went home, fed critters, and drove directly to Alec's birthday party…without daddy.

Ward's had uncontrolled bleeding from his nose/graft area because of the Coumadin, dangerously low blood pressure, dangerously high blood sugar (they've started him on insulin), severe dehydration, and narrowly missed getting a transfusion.

We're all exhausted and discouraged and just trying to make it through next Monday when they do the heart echo to see if that clot's gone. If it is, we'll be headed back to Houston to see about a (third) grafting.

10 March 2010 at 10:05am

We didn't go to the ER, but he did bleed all night and I've got a call into his heart doctor. His system flat cannot sustain another bleeding episode like this—it's a constant drip and it's been 16 hours again now.

They can't cauterize or even apply needed pressure—it's not a *hole* per se—the entire surface of that socket is like a sieve, and where it's coming from is both his nostril and the graft area. It's all connected via his sinuses, and there's still skin over the surface, so where it's bleeding from is several inches behind that—and they don't want to pack it because they'll tear up what's left of the graft and make it worse.

I need coffee. I'm afraid it's gonna be a long day...

10 March 2010 at 7:18pm

Okie dokie. We're home. Blood work still looks sort of ok—his red blood cell count is lower than it was on Friday, which was still below normal because of the LAST bleedy incident, and they said if he bleeds again he will need a transfusion.

So he's under strict NO BLEEDING orders.

I'm tired. He's exhausted.

Joe supervised school and took Alec to art class.

Joe Rocks.

12 March 2010 at 10:58pm

Maintaining so far. Blood pressure and blood sugars behaving, and there's been no more bleeding—although he looks horrifying because he's afraid to move, sit, stand, eat, wash, etc., so Tuesday's bandages are all still in place (including the very attractive TP wad up his nose). The very real concern is that if he removes the bandages, the really hard-won clots will come too and he'll start bleeding again.

The heart doctor said no more Coumadin, so he's been off that since Monday night—tomorrow we're going to VERY CAREFULLY try to get him cleaned up some...

13 March 2010 at 9:11am

So far today, the nostril packing (ok—toilet paper) fell out of its own accord last night, as did the pad over his graft area. So far so good, although he's not making any sudden moves...

16 March 2010 at 9:22am

The heart doctor says NO MORE CLOT and strongly recommends the plastic surgeon at MDAnderson fix "those holes in your head" ASAP. Like, pack the car and leave NOW.

Which is exciting, wonderful news and I left a message on the plastic surgery nurse's voicemail as soon as we left the cardio guy's office and emailed the plastic surgery PA as soon as we got home last night—we should hear something from them today re: scheduling.

He only sees patients in-clinic on Mondays and Wednesdays and I'm pretty sure he'll want a scan first, so it'll be next week anyway, which is fine since the Houston Livestock Show is on till Sunday night and you can't get a hotel room within 50 miles while that mess is going on.

We left the cardio guy's office at 3pm.

By 8pm Ward's gout was back and he's been confined to bed ever since.

Five. Freakin'. Hours. Of feeling good.

20 March 2010 at 12:47am

Ok. We're here in Houston (actually The Woodlands—about 30 miles north of Houston).

We have a tae kwon do tournament tomorrow, then we're just chillin' till Monday when Ward has to be at MDAnderson for:

-Blood work
-Chest x-ray
-EKG
-Consult with the doctor who will adjust all his meds in preparation for his
-Pre-op appointment with the surgeon on the 31st
-Surgery April 5th

Wheeeeeeeeeee...............................

20 March 2010 at 10:09pm

Alec Dixon—2nd degree level 1 black belt, competing against all levels of 2nd and 3rd degree black belts—bronze medal in traditional form, bronze medal in sparring, gold medal in freestyle form.

We've had Mexican food and are now chillaxin' in the hotel room watchin' Dirty Jobs.

23 March 2010 at 10:58pm

Sorry—had to play a full day of catch-up, not very successfully. I now have two briefcases and two laptop computers sitting right here next to me—one set for the tae kwon do club (I'm the treasurer) and one from my "real" job waiting for me to do a mess of stuff here at home tomorrow, my regularly scheduled day off.

Yippee.

Yesterday went pretty well. The internist who works at MDA and does the official script-check/adjustment pre-surgery and the final clearing of the patient was concerned about "something" he heard in Ward's left carotid artery, so we've got an appointment day after tomorrow here in Tyler for a Doppler echo on that. If it's blocked, they'll have to deal with THAT before surgery.

Sheesh.

So our schedule now stands as:

Thursday- Doppler echo of carotid artery, to be faxed immediately to the internist at MDA.

Next Wednesday (the 31st)- The surgeon at 8am, the internist at 10am, and the anesthesiologist somewhere that day.

The following Monday (the day after Easter)- surgery.

27 March 2010 at 9:35am

No word about the reading of the echo on the carotid yet.

We're basically ignoring all the health mess this weekend.

Today Ward and Alec are going to a board breaking clinic at tae kwon do, then lunch and the bookstore, while Joe and I pick up a tiller so we can get our tiny garden plot turned over here. This is something I've resisted the last few years. I've been doggedly planting at the new place and muttering, "We WILL be moved here before the end of planting season"—and losing every garden over there to reality. So this year we're planting here and planting small, and I'll just have to get over it as gracefully as I can (insert hysterical laughter from anyone who knows me).

The little local organic nursery is having their Spring Festival and Sale today, so we'll head over there later.

Tomorrow we're having Easter dinner since on Easter proper we'll be packing up and headed to Houston for surgery.

Maybe.

29 March 2010 at 11:31pm

Finally heard back from the heart doctor—carotids are less than 50% blocked (and she said that like it's a good thing?) so he's a go for surgery.

After planting the garden and packing up tomorrow, we're headed south...

31 March 2010 at 6:01pm

"You have two appointments today, and then we'll see you back here on Monday for surgery."

Medical translation:

"You have two appointments today, then we'll follow up with four appointments tomorrow because your blood work is still wonky—blood is too thin yet and your liver values are off."

Luckily, we've been around THIS block enough that I always pack that extra set of undies for everyone and bring enough cash for "just in case."

I'm going to miss payroll tomorrow for the first time ever—the three times in eight years that I've needed to be away, I've always anticipated and made arrangements for the bookkeeper to do it. So I've got 12 employees who will get a really un-funny April Fool...

It's a really pretty day here in Houston, so after our last appointment today we headed for Hermann Park and the Japanese Garden—all the azaleas and wisteria are out already.

I actually managed to get sunburned.

Wednesday, March 31, 2010

The Fable of the Baby Turtle

Once upon a time, a family was out walking in the park. It was a sunny warm day, and the azaleas and wisteria were blooming in reckless abandon in the absolute tidiness of the Japanese Garden.

Rounding a shady bamboo-lined corner, suddenly they were in front of a beautiful pond lined with flowers, burbling from a waterfall, flashing bright orange and white with the koi trolling just under the surface. Turtles of every size bathed in the sunshine draped over logs, rocks, and lily pads.

Just by chance, the mother looked down—and there at her feet was a baby turtle. It was determinedly traveling in the exact wrong direction and was heading for the shrubberies instead of the water. Gently she picked it up. She noticed how very dry it was—the heat of the sun was making the little shell brittle and the skin on its head and feet was flaking from lack of moisture.

After they carefully examined and admired the tiny reptile, she directed her son to place it into the water, where it paddled off happily.

Offhandedly, the mother said, "It better look out or it'll be lunch for a big fish."

This upset the boy, who questioned the wisdom of putting the turtle in the pond if there was a chance it would be eaten.

The family sat in the dappled shade of the wisteria trellis and gazed at the fountain in the middle of the pond.

While the safety of the shrubberies was almost certain to be free of large fish who might swallow the turtle, the sunshine and heat would've been its sure undoing—100% chance of non-survival.

In the water, there was the very real possibility of becoming a dinner item for the koi, or a duck, or even another really big turtle, but the pond is where the turtle belonged, where it was meant to be, and what it was adapted for. The only place the turtle had a chance of living at all was full of potential danger.

The apparent lack of obvious danger does not make a place safe if you're not meant to live there. Better to find your place in the world and deal with dangers as they come using your innate strengths as protection.

The turtle blink blink blinked, the water cascaded off of its sleek little shell, and it dove under a lily pad.

02 April 2010 at 1:20am

Home for a whole freakin' 72 hours. We got to the hospital at 7am and left at 4:30pm—just in time for rush hour.

The verdict: Blood work showed his clotting factors are steadily (if slowly) improving, most likely from the long time he's been on Coumadin. He's to take three days' worth of TINY bits (5mg) of Vitamin K, and before they do surgery on Monday they'll give him plasma.

He's still got some liver issues, but not enough to cancel surgery— just something (else) to watch...forever.

Tomorrow I need to do payroll (a day late) by noon, do some shopping and errands in the afternoon, more of the same Saturday, plus try to finish planting the garden, then clean guinea pig cages, pack suitcases, and get out the door 3pm Sunday....

They said to expect surgery to be about 9-10 hours on Monday, and about a week in hospital.

I'm headed for cocoa, then bed.

Maybe even in that order.

05 April 2010 at 12:15am

We're here in Houston and the alarm is set for 4am.
Report time to the hospital is 6am.
Surgery time is 7:30am.
Estimated time in surgery: TEN HOURS.

I hate this part.

05 April 2010 at 4:06pm

THE WARDSTER IS OUT OF SURGERY.

They did have to transfuse, but think he won't need ICU—we're
supposed to be able to see him in an hour or so.

I'll catch ya'll later- I'm headed to get Alec, a big M&M cookie,
and then we're going to see daddy.

Monday, April 5, 2010

When Even the Queen of the Universe Can't Fix It

It's now 11:27pm, and I've been up since 4am.

At 4am, my family got up, showered, and headed to MDAnderson Cancer Center for our 6am check in time for my husband's most recent surgery.

For eight years—over half the time we've been together as a couple, and for most of our son's life—my husband has been fighting with cancer and the after-effects of that, plus heart disease and diabetes.

We've had mostly good medical staff, some outstandingly brilliant medical staff, and just a few dismally inept medical staff, and I've learned something vitally important in all this:

Medical staff is human.

They have many patients and must attend to technical important things like dosages, reactions, and proper protocol. There's not much time left in their day to consider that every body they tend is also a husband, mother, child, grandparent.

Patients are more than organisms in need of healing—they are cherished members of family circles.

In what continues to be touted as the best health care nation in the world, every patient needs—not as in, "This sure would be nice", but as in, "If the patient does not have this he/she may die"—to have a patient advocate who is not afraid to ask questions, not afraid to speak up if something seems "off," and who is Family. Because no one cares for each patient as passionately as a family member.

Tonight, by chance, on our way out the door, I happened to overhear the nurse say she had been given orders to administer Tylenol to my husband for pain. He's in the beginning stages of liver disease and should NOT take Tylenol. Ever. That was confirmed by blood work taken here, at this hospital—truly one of the best in the world—less than four days ago. I alerted the post-op nurse of this and she changed his medication instructions accordingly. If I hadn't been there, my already weak and compromised husband would've been given a whoppin' dose of the very medication that has wreaked havoc on his liver.

But I digress...

My darling was wheeled out of pre-op at 8am, headed for his third total grafting in less than four years. In between blood clots in his heart and having to go on insulin for his diabetes, today they did a total new graft on the area where they removed cancer (three times). Only one graft was done post-cancer. These last two have failed due to healing issues.

That area is up on his head where his right eye used to be. It's been microsurgeried, enucleated, radiated, re-surgeried, and now grafted three times.

They've taken donor tissue (muscles and vessels) from his neck all three grafts, from his forearm once, his side under his other arm once, and this time from the leg that wasn't already harvested for veins they needed for his open heart surgery almost 15 years ago, plus skin grafts now 4 times.

And every time he goes in with resignation I cannot believe and bravery I cannot fathom.

He keeps on not for himself—this is a man who never asks for anything, ever—but for us, his wife and his son, and we spend the entire time he's asleep, and in recovery, and till he's healed, willing the medical staff to take care of him and willing him to be strong.

This time he was in surgery from about 9am till about 4pm, and had a more difficult time with recovery than the other times—he wasn't moved to a regular room till after 10pm. We're relieved that he didn't need to go to ICU even though he needed a transfusion for bleeding during surgery.

Many, many people—the family and friends of all of today's surgical patients—crowded the surgical waiting room today, starting all at 6am. By noon, about half of them were gone, and by

4 most of the rest were gone. Only a few of us were left then—the ones whose precious family members were undergoing "extensive procedures." Ward was one of the last out of the recovery room.

I'm exhausted. Our son is exhausted. I know my husband is exhausted. We all just want to go home now, be a normal family, and do normal stuff.

But we haven't had that careless scenario for a very long time.

The spectre of illness hangs heavy over our heads and it makes me crazy with worry, with frustration, with white hot anger at this curse on a man who deserves it less than any human I've ever met.

So we're here—ripped up by our roots from our beloved Pineywoods and thrust face-first into downtown Houston for the duration and many, many re-checks to follow. In the last four years we've gone no longer than four months without a trip down here for one appointment or another.

As I'm typing, I just now told my son to close up his computer and try to get to sleep—he was playing a computer game with almost frenetic intensity after spending 15 hours cooped up in a cancer hospital. His computer was not fully closed before his eyes were, and he's already sound asleep.

I'm headed to bed as soon as I make myself some tea, or maybe cocoa. I've spent all day trying to think of something to write here—something clever, or thoughtful, or important.

But in the end, this is it—what our family has learned at the expense of a "normal" life—when even the Queen of the Universe can't fix whatever's wrong, the only thing left is to love each other with a little more fervor, cherish each minute you can, reach out and touch a loved one, be patient, and kind, and selfless.

Petty arguments and disagreements are time-stealers, and we're all allotted a finite amount of minutes—grudges and revenge are abominations.

Tomorrow begins another round of recovery for my husband. Closing my eyes, all I can see are his poor ravaged features. Opening my eyes, I gaze on my sleeping 10-year-old boy who's seen much more physical horror than most adults.

And yet they both look to me for strength—when the truth is, my strength is a reflection of their character.

Love each other. Be strong for each other. Cherish each other.

I am the Queen of the Universe and I so decree.

06 April 2010 at 8:13pm

Hmmmm. Houston, we have a problem.

Ward's in pain. A lot of pain. And has been since he woke up from surgery.

Which is weird since the surgeon was so hopeful that this surgery would make his pain LESS, and not...WORSE.

They had him on the highest dose of morphine they could, and the morphine generally holds him fine and happy, but he was pawing at his head and literally trying to crawl out of the pain last night and this morning. I've never seen him in this much pain. Ever.

The surgeon came this morning and said, "Wow. Send for the pain management doctor."
The pain management doctor said, "Wow. Here—I'll order you a different narcotic right away."

That was at 2pm.

Alec wanted to go to the Natural Science museum during free admission times, which are 2-5 on Tuesdays, so we left and came back.

They were just delivering the new meds.

THREE HOURS LATER.

Said it was some sort of pharmacy hang-up, so I'll be killing me some pharmacists tomorrow.

This new stuff—relative of morphine, starts with a "D"—is working. Within an hour he was looking relaxed and sleeping.

So we're back at the hotel and eating delivery pizza.

For some reason Alec and I are still exhausted...

07 April 2010 at 9:13pm

Worked my way up through the pharmacy, leaving bleeding bodies hither and yon, till I got to the Inpatient Pharmacy Supervisor, who agreed wholeheartedly that filling an order for intense pain narcotics should be done in less than FOUR FREAKIN' HOURS. Supposedly he's looking into it and taking corrective action. Whatever. If you don't say anything, they can't fix a problem.

Then I had the pain management doctor come up to talk to me. Seems that on top of the Dilaudid, which is several times stronger than morphine and with a sedative property to boot, they have been continuing giving him his Neurontin—the medication he's been taking for nerve pain that PUTS HIM TO SLEEP when he takes it three times a day at home.

PROBLEM...????

After the first withheld dose of Neurontin, he was coherent for the first time since surgery. He hadn't eaten, stood up, anything since surgery two days ago because he's been zonked outta his mind or in tortured pain.

THEN I had the nurse page the on-call surgeon for the reconstructive dept. He was the assisting doctor during Ward's surgery. He said that yes, as a matter of fact, they did cause "significant surgical insult" to a bunch of previously un-injured nerves, but they hope that once the "initial insult pain" subsides, they'll not, yanno, keep him in head- splitting excruciating agony.

Golly, I hope he's right.

08 April 2010 at 9:10am

He's got the "magic button" and has been pushing it every time the green light flashes—every 10 minutes.

It was pushing morphine when that's what they had him on. Now it's the Dilaudid. I know it's a fine line—if he's got to be asleep to not hurt, fine. But he's also got to be awake enough to relay how he's feeling, order something to eat, and then be awake enough to eat it, and start walking to avoid other complications.

I'm fixin' to call up there right now—although I've learned, sadly, that even in the best hospital in the world, when some nurses say "He's resting comfortably," that means only that he's not screaming and bothering everyone.

(Yes. I've got some issues with Nurse Betty from yesterday that I'll be addressing today...)

08 April 2010 at 10:40am

Conversation with nurse just now—not Nurse Betty, but one who obviously did NOT get much info FROM Nurse Betty when the shifts changed—

"How's Ward today?"
"Fine—up in his chair and resting comfortably."
"Does he seem more alert than yesterday?"
"Oh yes. He's got his eye open and can answer questions."
"Is he eating? Drinking? Walking? Putting whole sentences together?"
"Umm. No. In fact, when I helped him into his chair, he kept grabbing at the air and trying to roll up his IV lines."
"Is his eye still rolling back into his head, and does it take several times asking him simple questions to get an answer?"
"Yes."
"When he finally does answer, do his answers make any damn sense at all?"
"Well...not really."
"Then he's not any better than yesterday."
"I guess not."

08 April 2010 at 8:08pm

Well. It's official. Ward's mind is taking a little break from his body.

They're not sure if it's a lovely 60's mix of residual anesthetic, morphine, Dilaudid, and the other various pain meds, or if there's something actually going on physically, but my normally mild-mannered, best-patient-in-the-world husband is fractious, paranoid and argumentative.

He's confused, but knows he's confused, which just really pisses him off.

He is sure the nurses are all out to get him, sneaking up on him, and wanting to kill him.

When he recognizes me, he either begs me not to leave because he's sure he'll die if I'm not there, or accuses me of ordering the hospital staff to torture him.

He didn't believe me when I told him today is Thursday.

He didn't know he is at MDAnderson.

He can't remember what year it is, begged the nurses not to put him on the boat (?), and keeps either trying to pull out all his IV's, drains, and stitches, or reaching for some imaginary critters flying at his head.

He insisted on holding my hand, then freaked out because he thought he'd grown an extra appendage.

One of the doctors came in and asked Ward, "Who's this pretty lady sitting next to you?" (Meaning me).

Ward looked from me to him several times before frowning and petulantly telling the doctor, "That's a meerkat." Apparently he thought he was being kept company by a huge African rodent wearing bi-focals.

This had all better be wildly hilarious someday...

They had a psychiatrist talk to him and he said, "Wow. He's really stoned, huh?"

They've ordered blood work to see if his electrolytes are off and a CT scan just to rule out if the cause is actually physical—a vessel seeping into his brain (which would explain why he was so HORRIBLY painful right out of surgery), or had a stroke during surgery or something—but they can't do anything to him. He won't let them. It took me an hour to talk him into taking his pain pill. He said it was poison.

They don't want to give him any more pain stuff IV or sedate him and add anything more to the mix he's already got going.

Alec's been with a friend of ours all day, but by 5pm Alec was ready to go back to the hotel, so they called a sitter to stay with Ward to make sure Ward doesn't, you know, as he keeps saying, "Get the fuck out of here."

That is not a word normally in his vocabulary.

08 April 2010 at 9:48pm

Ward just demanded that the nurse call me so I could reassure him that the pills she wanted to give him are not, in fact, poison.

Then he gave me no end of shit about not being there with him.

Then he told me under no circumstance was I to bring Alec up there while he's all fucked up.

Then he yelled, "WHY AREN'T YOU **HERE**?"

Then he fell asleep and dropped the phone into his lap.

It's gonna be a loooooooong night...

08 April 2010 at 10:12pm

They're TRYING to check everything but he won't let them near him.

I talked him into taking the Narcol (?) for pain, his regular anti-depressant, and some Seratol (?) to relax him, and he seemed better after just a little bit.

They're hoping that letting all the IV stuff work its way out of his system will calm him down enough where they can do a full blood workup, including electrolytes and a CT scan, to rule out a physical cause.

09 April 2010 at 10:14am

I talked to the nurse a little while ago. Ward's no better.

I've called his brothers to come down so someone he knows is always with him. There was hesitation and I tearfully (because I'm exhausted and NEED HELP, DAMMIT) reminded them I've never asked them to come help with anything, ever, before this.

I've called a friend of ours, whom Alec considers his brother, to come keep Alec company.

I went to bed last night at 10pm.

Why am I still so tired?

09 April 2010 at 6:54pm

Ok. The BEST news is that the CT scan and blood work shows
there's no physical cause.
So he's just batshit crazy, which should wear off with a nice dose
of withdrawal over the next few days.

It was discouraging to find him WORSE this morning—he's now
restrained to the bed. He does a lot of growling at people, but
hasn't actually bitten anyone, although he did threaten the male
nurse with physical violence (anyone who knows Ward even a
little bit knows how out of character THAT is). They tell me that
he's much better when I'm around, so I can't imagine how he's
acting otherwise.

So, good news—our friend Jordan is already on his way and will
be here about 9pm to pick up Alec. He's taking him up to his
sister's house in Spring (about an hour north of here) where they'll
spend the night and go to the Crawfish Festival tomorrow. This
frees me to go back to the hospital and spend the night with
Ward—his brothers are 'having a hard time making it work" to
come down here—they've both got previous plans. (Insert
whatever descriptive curse words you can think of here. I did).

Hopefully he'll be lucid enough for Alec to accompany me on
Sunday since the kids' room is closed.

Physically, he's perfect—healing well and not infected. So once he
gets rid of the Crazy, he should be good to go.

09 April 2010 at 9:29pm

I'm just waiting for Alec's ride to get here and then I'm on my way
back to the hospital.

Jordan just called for directions and said he'd keep Alec tomorrow night too if Ward's still living in Crazytown.

10 April 2010 at 1:49pm

I'm back at the hotel after spending the night at the hospital. I had to get a little sleep, a shower, do the laundry since we're officially out of underwear right now, and have something to eat since the last thing I had was 8pm last night. And that was Sunchips and the head of a chocolate rabbit.

Ward's doing better. He's a lot better as of last night.

I walked in the room and there was Ward looking back at me for the first time since surgery over five days ago. No restraints. No growling. No cursing.

I spent the night with him, along with the sitter he's assigned since he still wants to get up and wander and forgets about his drains and IV, and though he rested a bit, he hasn't had any good, sound sleep since surgery—he's exhausted.

He ate a few bites of pudding last night and one bite of eggs this morning, but otherwise hasn't had anything to eat since before surgery, so he's gotta be lightheaded.

At 3am he HAD to get up and walk, so the nurse (last night's nurse and sitter were both angels pure and truly) let him get up and helped him walk for the first time since surgery. He did two laps around the floor holding onto his IV stand and was able to work off some nervous energy. Then they got him a bath and tucked him in and he was able to relax for about an hour before starting to fidget again.

In a spectacular display of dexterity, right at shift change at 7am, he went from lying flat on his back "reading," to on all fours to standing upright ON THE BED. Then did a very passable hostage-taker impression of hollering to the (ya think?) many concerned hands on him trying to keep him from falling, "EVERYBODY JUST BACK OFF. STOP PUSHING ME!"

He finally heard my voice through it saying, "Dear, just sit on the bed there right where you are." He said he wanted to sit on the chair I'd been in. I said,"Ok, but you must sit on the bed first". He asked why. I said, "Because you can't FLY."

He thought about it for a minute...then, "Oh. OK". And sat down.

My guess is that set his "ready for discharge" time back a good 12 hours or so...

He's still fuzzy, still foggy, still seeing things not visible to those of us not in the same plane of reality that he's in—ants on the floor, worms on the page of his book, and thinking the bed is tilting— still not sure of where he is or why he's there or why he can't go home, but for the most part he's sweet funny Ward again.

Golly I've missed him

10 April 2010 at 10:29pm

Ya. So.

Since Ward's no-account brothers are no-shows via voicemail because of "previous family commitments" (I'm sorry—what the hell is WARD?) I left him for FOUR HOURS this morning.

I left him almost lucid and easy to talk to, and came back to...a raving maniac.

Apparently, the nurse tried to give him his pills to swallow, and he refused. He's been taking them in pudding without incident which SHOULD have been on his chart or at least relayed from one shift to the next.

She thought he was in pain.

So she dosed him with some IV Dilaudid.

Square Freakin' One.

The only reason he escaped being restrained is because I got there just before the exploding point, although he was clearly more than "agitated." And even though they say he's better when I'm there than not, it didn't mean he didn't still turn on me several times, and on the nurses more than once—especially sweet little Sheila, who he was convinced was a nefarious cad named Derek. He told me he wanted me to call Joe and have him come down and shoot off Derek's pinky toe.

To say I "had words" with everyone involved is the understatement of the century, and after almost a week of this and being so close to having him back I was in tears as well.

So he got the Dilaudid, then they undid his IV because he was so fractious, which meant he wasn't peeing it out of his system, so it just percolated the whole time I was gone.

I called Jordan, who is keeping Alec another night, and my friend Cathy (the same friend who FLEW down the day after being on a 14 day road trip to be with me for his first surgery so very long ago) and she's taking the day off of work Monday and driving down from Dallas tomorrow after church to be with Alec tomorrow afternoon/evening and Monday. It's not a total waste for her—she'll spend the night with her son, daughter-in-law, and new grandbabies tomorrow night.

It was just the one dose, so by the time I left to change clothes and get something to eat, eight hours after getting it, he's not quite where he was this morning, attitude-wise, but after I reassured him that I'm not going HOME, just two miles to the hotel to change and eat, then come right back, (OK, I left out that I'm fixin' to get a nap, too...) he said "OK- bring me back some cocoa."

Can do, Big Fella. Can do.

11 April 2010 at 9:15pm

Hey. Lookit who's here—it's Ward.

As of 11:30 this morning he was back—fuzzy but not irritated—and totally exhausted.
He was very anxious last night when I returned less than two hours after leaving—the nurse had been trying to give me time to nap, so when he started asking to call and talk to me 15 minutes after I left (something I TOLD her to let him do) she said "I'm sorry, Mr. Dixon, all we have is her cell phone number and that's long distance from here—we can't call that from the floor".

He didn't think that that meant our cell phone has a different area code from Houston; he took that to mean *I* was far away—that I'd left him here.

When I got back he was almost in tears and I had to sleep in the bed with him. He finally slept really and truly, but every 20 minutes or so would startle and I'd rub his back and tell him I was right there and he'd go back to sleep immediately.

I stayed in hospital till after the consult with Symptom Management—now his primary care doctor—who has officially put Dilaudid as a life-threatening allergy in the computer so it comes up bright red on everything. She prescribed something for his throat, which hurts more than his surgical sites from yelling and open mouth sleeping in addition to the breathing tube irritation from surgery. And something to really truly take the edge off his anxiety at losing so many days and let him get some real, good, sleep.

We gently caught him up to date—he, of course, is "just waking up from surgery," so it was kind of a shock to him that it's not Tuesday but Sunday. He remembers a lot of the hallucinations— the UFO with the gun turret, the bugs and weird animals everywhere, and some of the imaginary people he thought were out to get him.

I went over his group of "good" people for the day—the nurse, the doctor, the sitter who he thought was the nefarious Derek yesterday—just in case seeing them gives him the heebie jeebies, and he wrote down their names.

I started telling him some of the funny stuff he did and he laughed at it all—even his Mooning of the Entire 11th Floor episode.

I told him I'd be back tonight with Alec for a little while, and that Alec and I have to spend the night in the hotel for the rest of our time here, but that his son and I will never, ever, ever leave Houston without him. Ever.

Then I somehow made it to the hotel without incident and totally fell apart. Yanno how, when a loved one is sick, you think "if I could take the pain, I would?" Apparently that works, because by the time I laid my head on the pillow, I had a splitting headache and wasn't making any damn sense at all. I thought things were pushing against the back of my pillow. I saw stuff up on the wall.

It'd been since Thursday night that I'd slept more than an hour or two at a stretch and the most nutritious thing I'd eaten were parts of a chocolate rabbit. I've spent all that time with Ward, being literally crushed at the unnecessary setback he had, and pushing so very hard to make sure he got what he needed.

My friend Cathy got here, made coffee since part of my headache was that I hadn't had any caffeine today, and made me lie in bed in the dark while I babbled.

Jordan returned Alec, and Alec left with Cathy while I slept until they came back with real food for dinner—Alec had her go to the Chinese restaurant where he remembered every one of my favorite things. He's taking very good care of me.

I'm fixin' to take a shower, 'cause I'm mostly fine and really need one, and if I'm STILL fine afterwards, Alec and I will go up to visit Ward for a little bit before coming back here—I promised both of them I would. I'll call up there and really talk to Ward first to be sure there haven't been any...setbacks.

Check under yer pillows for monsters—they're there, I tells ya....

12 April 2010 at 11:10am

Ya. So about 9:30 last night I called Ward's room to make sure all was still fine before taking Alec up there and the nurse said "He's been fine all day but now won't take his meds and doesn't allow anyone near him."

I got a shower, still feeling dizzy, the headache barely held at bay by meds, and we went up there. He's completely paranoid again, but at least not hallucinating and not combative. He gave us both a huge hug and wrote a note to me that there was poison in the jello.

I left Alec with him and went to talk to the nurse. Turns out the doctor did NOT prescribe what she said she would, and he'd gotten nothing for his throat or anxiety. I had the nurse page the doctor. I asked if Ward had wanted to call me and she said no.

I asked the sitter if he'd wanted to call me and she said yes.

I told the nurse AGAIN that any time he wants to call me they need to LET HIM.

I told them point blank that I'm VERY discouraged that every time I leave there he seems better, and when I return he's worse again because of something that they directly did or didn't do.

I told Ward that I had to get Alec back to the hotel cuz it was 10pm and that I still had a headache and needed to get to bed and he understood.

By the time I got back to the hotel, I was so sick with headache I was *just* this side of vomiting as I hit the bed, where I remained till 6am.

I'm still woozy, but I called Ward and told him I'd be up this afternoon for a little while. Bless his heart, even all fuzzy and paranoid his first concern is that I'm OK and need to get better.

I talked to the day nurse, and she said THIS MORNING (prolly after the page jogged her memory) the doctor called in something for the throat and anxiety and they should be delivered shortly.

Honestly, right now his main problems are that his sore throat is making him unable to eat, which is making him lightheaded, and lack of sleep, which is making him paranoid and loopy.

If they can fix THAT, I think we'll be golden.

I'm going to see if I can roll a few heads over the phone, too—that always cheers me up

12 April 2010 at 7:37pm

Ward sounds better on the phone, which is the only place I've talked to him today. I keep thinking I really did absorb some of his pain, exhaustion, and Crazy, because I still can't function today without being nauseatingly dizzy. If that's true, I'm ok with it.

Alec broke his flip-flops, so we went to Target and got new ones. I was so dizzy I had to sit down while he chose them. He left his book in Cathy's car, so we went to Barnes and Noble and I stayed in the car with my eyes closed while he went in alone, found his book, and paid for it. The thought of dealing with the round-and-round parking garage and the elevators at the hospital were overwhelming and we barely got back to the hotel, where I collapsed onto the bed again.

Six hours later and I'm STILL dizzy. Dammit. We need to go to Kroger's and get some food, so I'll have to make myself do that—it's only about a mile, straight shot, so I think I can.

I did call Patient Advocacy and she was going to call the Head Nurse and have her call me, which she never did.

Ward does sound better and I talked to his sitter today, who ASKED ME what she could do to help all of us—much better. She even called when the psychiatrist was there so I could talk to him—much, much better.

He said that Ward's improved but still easily confused. I told him if we can get his throat where he can EAT and his brain where he can get good restful SLEEP, that would do the trick, and he agreed.

Ward's main concern is that *I'm* OK. He told me to stay in bed as long as needed. I asked how the staff is today and he said, "Fine." I asked if he's taking his pills and he sounded a little surprised and said, "Yes. Of course."

Our friend Martha, who works up there, stopped in to see him and called me to verify that he is in a much better mood.

If he continues to improve, I think they'll spring him Wednesday. Sure hope I can drive five hours home by then.

13 April 2010 at 1:52am

I passed from dizzy/nauseated to dizzy/vomiting as of 8pm. So I went to bed, where I've been fitfully dozing.

The phone just now rang. They have to take Ward back into surgery NOW. Tonight. Now.

The flap is not circulating blood anymore and is failing. How can he be there by himself??? I really can't stand this and can't see through the tears and dizziness. They're calling me to get my permission to send my poor, tired, already-compromised husband back into surgery.

I have no words for how scared I am right now.

I talked to Ward. He knows something is up, but not really. Dr. Hanasono promised me he wouldn't let anything happen to Ward, and Lord help him if it does.

If they can't save the flap, they'll have to remove it and just skin graft the socket—They don't have much hope that will heal, but right now there's no other option.

They don't even want me there just in case I'm really germ-sick and not fatigue-sick. He can't risk that too.

I feel totally helpless for the first time in my life.

13 April 2010 at 5:06am

The surgeon just called. Ward's out of surgery. They were able to
fix the flap. The surgeon said Ward hardly bled at all and his heart
stayed strong. He'll go to ICU and should be back in his room
before lunchtime. I've spent the last three hours crying.

Other than the people I've actually grown inside me and given birth
to, I've never loved anyone as fiercely as Ward.

When I talked to him before surgery I told him that I love him and
that I hate that I can't be at the hospital. I couldn't stop crying—he's
been through so much this week and was just now almost better,
but far from strong.

He said, "Hey, don't worry. It's OK. You take care of yourself and
get better. I'll be alright—we've got a lot to do yet."

Yes. Yes we do, my love.

13 April 2010 at 10:30am

Ya. I hadn't heard anything, so I called the floor.

No Ward.

I called ICU.

He's still there, but NOT expected is:

-He's still unconscious and on a ventilator.
-The last chest x-ray shows infection.

The nurse sounded so chipper and upbeat. She said, "We hope to
get him awake and breathing on his own by TOMORROW." I

made sure they all know **NO DILAUDID** and she said YES they know.

She said I can call up there to check on him whenever I want, but I can't be in hospital within 24 hours of vomiting.

I only vomited the once, at 8pm. That gives me today to stay in bed and get un-dizzy.

All night I couldn't stop thinking about my friend Sunni, who lost her Jim after he had a mild stroke, after which he got pneumonia and died. And my friend Sharlotte, who lost her Edward while they were doing a "routine" MRI after intestinal surgery and he aspirated and died. These were both in the last 6 months.

When the surgeon called at four to tell me he was done and the surgery was a success and he'd be back in his room by lunchtime, I slept for the first time, because everything was going to be ok.

Now I'm not so sure anymore.

*I just got an email reply from the surgeon's PA. Very quick response—less than 30 minutes. Of course the gist of my email to her was, "WHAT THE HELL????"

She said the x-ray was done after the surgeon talked to me. They wanted to be sure the breathing tube was in the right place. They left it in in case they have to put him back under with gas for pain control, as they're afraid to use opiates (duh). The ICU radiologist must've seen the infection. They're headed back up there as soon as the doctor finishes the appointment he's in and they'll call me when they get there and find out what's what.

Tuesday, April 13, 2010

When Just Being Thicker Than Water is No Damn Good At All

"Blood is thicker than water".

I never did know what the hell that was supposed to mean. I mean, first of all—duh.
Second of all, so what?

I've found that in a pinch, when push comes to shove, when your back's against the wall and when the shit hits the fan, merely being "thicker than water" doesn't cut the mustard. You need a rope, good and strong.

And in actual practice, most of those that could be defined as "thicker than water" have been about as useful as tits on a bull.

My folks have helped us out as they could, so they're excluded.

Ward's mom was an angel.

But by and large, when we've really needed help—and unfortunately that's been a frequent event—it's been our friends who've rushed forward to catch us, to hold us, to steady us, and keep us from going over the edge.

Years ago, we stopped depending on our blood relatives and started forming our "real" families of people we knew would be there for us.

That's not unusual. A lot of people do that. What is unusual is that, instead of banding together with others just like us, we made our "real" family out of people with an amazing combobulation of religions, genders, nationalities, races, orientations, ages, and political scope. I credit the interwebs with allowing us to meet such a glorious lot, although my innate oddness would've ensured that our manufactured immediate family would not resemble our neighbors at all, regardless.

Right now, my husband and his wife and son are in the most distress we've ever been in. He's in ICU at a huge cancer hospital and on a ventilator. He is not breathing on his own and is possibly in congestive heart failure.

Our home and farm are being cared for indefinitely by a huge bear of a man from Montana who's moved into our home and family. We've turned him into an old chicken herding hippie, and he's Friend to Ward, Uncle to Alec, and he has me packing a purse pistol named Thelma.

The friend our son thinks of as his brother drove down for the weekend and took Alec to NASA and a grand tour of the seedier parts of Houston.

My friend of over 30 years, who lives in the Dallas area, drove down after church to spend Sunday afternoon and evening with Alec.

Our friends who live in Houston are there always—on call—to take any or all of us out for distraction or into their home for comfort.

My home-school moms are coming here tomorrow to be here for us.

Alec has had offers literally from around the country by people who want to take him into their homes to protect him, love him, and support him while I deal with the mundane horrors of the cancer hospital.

Alec, Ward, and I have faced eight years of this mess together, and together we'll face this go-round. Together. We're not leaving here without my husband and Alec's daddy.

People call me and email me and message me from around the world. We're being prayed for, candles lit, energies and jujus sent, and all gods and spirits called for strength for my family.

Friends we've met, hugged in real life, and those we haven't, from sea to shining sea, both new and one I've known for 35 years, are there at the touch of a mouse, or the tapping out of a phone number.

We feel their love as a shawl around our shoulders—warm and sheltering.

Our friends ARE our Family—better than some sticky ooze that's claim to fame is being "thicker than water." Our friends are our rope, and we cling tightly to them while being beaten down by the storms of illness. Over and over and over again.

They are stalwart. And true. And without them, we'd have drowned long ago.

13 April 2010 at 1:33pm

The surgeon just called. He does NOT have an infection, but every time they try to take him off the ventilator, he stops breathing.

He's not breathing.

They suspect heart failure.

The cardio guys are coming in to see for sure. The blood guy is coming in to test to see if clotting is happening for some other reason and causing the problem.

The cardio guys want him asleep so he rests. The brain guys want him awake because the longer he's asleep, the longer it'll take him to recover mentally.

Again.

I may be running a little fever now and my intestines are giving me trouble, so they won't let me in there even if I could drive.

No one has said "this is it," but...

Please please please—

I really can't stand any more.

13 April 2010 at 7:43pm

The heart guys have put him on something and want to give it till morning to get his heart as strong as possible before trying to wake him up again.

They said he's stable.

Our friend Martha went to see him on her break and she told him we're here and not going anywhere without him.

Two of my home-school mom friends are coming down in the morning and will stay at least a few days.

I showered and ate some soup, walked to the laundry room (funny how even in crisis the underwear doesn't wash itself), and was dizzy again by the time I walked back, so I think I'll let his brothers be the heroes tonight and go up there. I'll try tomorrow.

His brothers are here because I called them and told them how very seriously ill and fragile he is and I suggested they come see him.

They said they'd "see what they could do" and I came completely unhinged.

I told them point blank that Ward—their BROTHER—could die. Soon. Now. And that for the love of all that's holy they were to get their asses in the car and head this way NOW.

So they did. 'Bout fucking time.

I've been calling Ward every few hours—the ICU nurse holds the phone to his ear—and this last time I said, "Yanno, I'm just gonna bug you till you wake up, so you may as well just get on with it."

I know he can hear me.

I know the sound of my voice is something he can hang on to.

13 April 2010 at 9:41pm

Ward's brothers are up there now. The only reason I know that is because I called them to help them navigate Houston and the hospital and they were already there...without calling me to say so.

Just doing the laundry—all one load of it—brought back my dizziness and the hint of a headache, so that puts the kibosh on going up there tonight.

Ward loves his brothers deeply.

I've been there for him for 15 years and am there now in heart, soul, and the end of the phone cord every few hours. Hard as it is, I think WARD needs this time with just his brothers.

I hope to hell they cherish it like I know he will.

13 April 2010 at 10:10pm

Alec's amazing.

There was one time, on Sunday night when he and I visited Ward, that he started breaking down. I asked him what was scaring him.

That daddy was crazy? No.

That mommy was sick? No.

That MOMMY was acting a little crazy, he's 10 and may be all alone in Houston with two batshit crazy parents? He teared up and nodded.

I showed him my cell phone—all the speed dial numbers of people who love him and would get on an airplane if necessary to make sure he's safe, always.

That gave him options. And power. And made it OK.

14 April 2010 at 2:34pm

I held my husband's hand for the first time since Sunday night a few hours ago.

Talked to the cardiologist—apparently, after this surgery, Ward's heart went wild and they thought he had a heart attack. All the tests point negative on that, which is not really comforting since I know that, while the heart can get stronger from an attack, failure is irreparable.

The next 48 hours will remain critical. He's in congestive heart failure and the clot is back in his heart—the doctor said from the calcification. He doubts it was completely gone. So they need to give IV nitroglycerin to calm his heart, and they need to give him enough IV Lasix to get the fluid out of his lungs, but not so much that they stop flow in the tiny brand new vessels they just attached in the new graft.

They can't even think of waking him up yet since he'll think he's drowning (and be right).

Yet another disconcerting thing—the cardiologist kept saying, "His x-rays here from '07 and '08 show no failure, so this must've been in the last year," thus assuming he went into the first surgery compromised.

He said all this while totally ignoring me and talking straight at the brothers, who were in the room too, and who nodded their heads sagely like they knew the first thing about Ward's medical history Finally I couldn't stand any more and interjected firmly but as politely as I could manage—

"NO. HE HAD A CHEST X RAY HERE LESS THAN A MONTH AGO. DID YOU LOOK AT **THAT** ONE???"

No. He had not.

Guess what? The x-ray taken one week before the April 5th surgery showed NO heart failure. None. Nada. Zip. Zero.

Meaning that the strain of two major surgeries in eight days, and MAINLY (in my humble know-nothing opinion) the six days of physical drain he had while they held him hostage in CrazyTown, caused heart failure.

So now he's very, very ill.

I'm more than a little annoyed.

His brothers saw him last night, and this morning, and, in the wake of "the next 48 hours are critical" pronouncement, are going home this afternoon.

They never asked how I'm doing. Or how Alec's doing. Or if we needed money. Or made a move to even touch me, let alone give me a hug. Or said anything like, "Hey—it's lunchtime. Before we go, let's take you and Alec out to eat since we're sure you know a good place."

I was gonna give them a quick primer on the workings of the parking token machines, which are nightmares, but decided to let them figure it out for themselves.

Bleah. Enough of that.

The GREAT NEWS is that, when I got there, I took Ward's hand and said, "It's me, honey. I'm right here with you. I'm better, and when I can't be right here, I'll still call and bug you every few hours on the phone. Alec and I aren't leaving Houston without you. It's your job to rest, get strong, and keep fighting, and my job to be here and give 'em all hell."

He squeezed my hand.

I told him, "Alec can't see you here in ICU, and so he opted to stay at the hotel by himself alone for the first time. I told him not to start anything on fire."

His one remaining eyebrow shot straight up in obvious alarm.

He's in there.

And lord help the hospital staff, I'm out here.

14 April 2010 at 11:18pm

Our home school friends got here late afternoon and took Alec to the grocery store while I went to see Ward again. No changes, although they placed a feeding tube, and I think he was pretty worn out. But, if I watched him closely, I could see his breathing change just a bit when I'd say certain things that he would've answered (if that makes sense).

We took our friends to dinner at Southwell's Grill—good burger joint—and now Alec is over in their room giving me some quiet time. Truth told, he's been an angel, and if I'm feeling bad, all I hear from him is the click of his computer keys. He's writing a Star Wars story. He's read a lot of the novels—from the adult science fiction section, not kids' books—which are about 400 pages each. He blows through one in a week.

The surgeon called, which he didn't have to do since Ward's pretty much been turned over to ICU for care. He gave me every update he's gotten, told me that he's got to be overseas from tomorrow till Monday—who'da thunk Ward would still be in hospital at this stage of the game, much less THIS?—But he was going to see him tomorrow morning, had given his staff directives to call him every day (including over the weekend) with updates, and will see him again first thing Monday morning.

He told me he feels strongly that they "should" be able to pull Ward thru this, but if one thing goes wonk-ier it'll be...tricky.

He told me to stay strong and keep rested because even in the best-case scenario this will be, "A very, very long haul to get him back."

He reminded me (although I didn't need reminding) that he's known us for almost four years and that he sees Ward's a little more tired and wore out every time he sees him. That the last (has it only been?) nine days have taken a horrific toll.

Best-case scenario at this point is 48 hours from now they'll try to back him off of the ventilator if he's strong enough.

Then if he does very well, another few days in ICU.

Then if he does very well, at least another week in hospital.

So best case scenario is another two weeks down here.

Of course, it could be months.

I told him I didn't care how long the haul was, as long as Ward's with us.

That Ward's son needs him.

That *I* need him.

While in the room with him, I played Ward's fingers over my ring finger—I'm wearing his wedding band right next to mine like I always do after his surgeries till I can put it back on his finger once he's awake—I told him those rings will stay right there next to each other till he and I are right next to each other again.

Thursday, April 15, 2010

Spare Me the Drama, Mama—I Crave Some Mundane

I vividly remember our most recent family hug.

It was Sunday night, four days ago now.

It was much like any other of a million family hugs—Ward, standing tall and strong, myself wrapped in his left arm, his son wrapped in his right—the three of us twined into a human pretzel held together with comfort, love, and familiarity.

We were only slightly inconvenienced by the IV's and drains attached to Ward, and the IV stand didn't get in our way at all.

It was a good hug. Nay, a great hug—filled with relief and exhaustion and joy all mingled together. Ward was absolutely and completely light-at-the-end-of-the-tunnel into healing after a very rocky week following what was supposed to be a pretty routine, albeit extensive, surgery.

Alec and I left the hospital feeling good, Ward went to bed feeling good—we all anticipated Ward's release from the hospital by Wednesday at the latest.

Wednesday. Yesterday.

I'd fallen asleep fitfully. I'd caught a bug in hospital after a week of worry and sleeplessness and eating sparsely and horribly, and was just then feeling the full effects—dizziness, nausea—when the phone brought me suddenly, adrenalin-ly, sickeningly awake at 1am.

Ward needed emergency surgery immediately. In the middle of the night. But they assured me it would be a quick fix and he'd be back in his room by lunchtime Monday.

It didn't work that way, and he's now lying in ICU attached to a ventilator and in congestive heart failure.

And I wonder whatever happened to "normal."

I asked my son yesterday if he could even, in his ten year existence, remember a time when our family life didn't consist of hospitals, operations, recovery, repeat. And though he made light of thinking it over, he was serious when he said, "No. Not really."

I'm trying to come to terms with our new reality. Not our beloved old knock-around house at the edge of Brownsboro TX (pop. 756)—chickens in the yard, turkeys on the porch, drifting off to sleep to the chorus of hundreds of spring peepers down by the pond—but this hotel room in the middle of Houston (4th largest city in the US of A), the non-stop cacophony of helicopters and ambulances rushing to the hospital district glowing just a few blocks away.

And, as crushing as living here with no set ending, no date we can circle on the calendar, is, we refuse to leave without Ward. He's here. We're here. They tell us it's going to be a "very, very long haul" but that's fine as long as we're all here and all together.

I've known Ward for 16 years and we've been a couple almost 15. This is not my first go-around on the relationship/marriage train, but this is the only time I can honestly say there's never been one minute, one second, that I've ever thought, "Hmmmm, this just isn't working out."

Ward's the best friend I've ever had, the best father I could ever imagine for Alec, and truly the Love of My Life. And even though I'm surly, argumentative, and difficult, for some reason he feels the same way about me.

But while other couples—even those who still love each other deeply—stagnate and flounder a bit under the day- to-day child raising and working and bill paying, wishing for some excitement to knock the dust off of their routines, we crave the opposite:

Quiet. Normal. Boring. Stay-at-home Life.

I know, from tuning into every morsel of his being, which is wrapped up, trussed up, invaded, and hooked to machines that surround him carnivorously, that he can hear me. I hold his hand, and talk to him, and at sensible times there are signs—the twitch of his hand in mine, the raising of an eyebrow, the flicker of an eyelid, the rising or lowering of his blood pressure—that tell me he's fighting as hard as he can. That no one wants to go home more than he does.

So we wait. And I keep him company, holding his hand and reading aloud to him in an almost insane caricature of normalcy. I pretend not to notice the nurses and others coming in and going about their medical business—the business of keeping my husband alive till his body is strong enough to once again keep itself alive.

And outside the hospital walls, I meet other people who complain petulantly about the irritating habits of spouses, or the boredom of their jobs, or the tiring, mind-numbing chores inherent in the raising and training of children, and they look at me like we're all in the same secret club and ask, "Yanno what I mean?"
I think of what I wouldn't give right now to find beard hairs in the bathroom sink, or a collection of half-empty soda cans abandoned around the house, or even to simply be at home in our own bed—together.

And I can't even feign thinking about it before answering, "No. Not really."

15 April 2010 at 7:49pm

Today I dealt with some work stuff, and some daily living stuff—arranging our living quarters for the duration.

Alec, April, Christine, and Hopie left before I did on a Museum Extravaganza Day, and I'm back at the hotel before they are.

I got to the hospital about noon, and was able to talk to the ICU doctor who will be Ward's monitor till Monday morning. She was cautiously optimistic.

-The Lasix is working, so the fluid is leaving his lungs—good.

-They can't place a working feeding tube due to how swollen his poor throat is—bad.
-His heart is behaving without nitroglycerin—good.
-Due to the heart failure, it's still not pumping worth a dang—bad.
-The graft is still viable, and all the pathology on the "stuff" they took out came back negative—good.
-They plan on him staying on the ventilator another WEEK or so— bad.

So, sort of the same—a few things better, some not progressing as hoped.

Last night I told him, "I'll bring a book tomorrow and start reading to you," and then thought,"Hey! What happened to his stuff from the regular room???" and went upstairs to retrieve it. It's not there. No one knows where it is. So today I spent three hours trying to track it down—mainly his GLASSES and BOOKS, to no avail.

Finally, someone said, "I'll call Patient Advocacy," and I rolled my eyeballs and told them that I'd called them for some other concerns LAST WEEK and had not heard back, even though I'd called again Monday. The Patient Advocacy supervisor is supposed to call me tomorrow.

So I spent a good several hours with Ward, reading to him. I re-started a book he'd just given me. We had discussed during his few lucid moments last week how much I was enjoying it, and he just was so tickled. He'd said he knew I'd like it, that's why he got it— and he smiled that wonderful loving smile.

Therefore, I decided to share the whole thing with him, since we seem to have plenty of "down time" ahead of us.

When I started reading, his blood pressure upper reading was about 160. After just a few minutes, it dropped to 140, only shifting up again when the nurse came and interrupted us with checks and procedures.

Before opening the book, I told him what the doctor had said—that he's better today than yesterday, and he needs to keep fighting—and his hand twitched in mine.

And so I read-

"Where Bigfoot Walks: Crossing the Dark Divide" by Robert Michael Pyle

Chapter One—Not Looking for Bigfoot

"Sometimes the things you believe in become more real to you than all the things you can explain away or understand." - Tommy Albright in Lerner and Lowe's Brigadoon....

16 April 2010 at 7:33pm

I spent the morning doing work stuff and laundry, the afternoon reading to Ward, and am now making sammmiches to meet 'n eat with Christine and Alec before seeing *Cats* on-stage in Hermann Park.

The Lasix did its job. Ward peed out two liters of lung fluid yesterday, and today they worked to slowly bring him just far enough out of sedation to wiggle toes on command, but not so much that he'll fight the ventilator or hurt. They are also starting intravenous feedings tonight to get his strength back.

As he's coming awake, his blood pressure and heart are reacting—remember, he is not even aware he went BACK to surgery. What a shock THIS will be, both mentally and physically.

So he's back on nitro and IV blood pressure meds.

Baby steps...baby steps.

He frowned when they pricked his finger for his blood sugar test and gave me a "closed eye wink" when I kissed his forehead.

I left him with this imagery from the book I'm reading:

"In the early morning I walked back to the first mossy brook, on the Quartz Creek Trail to filter a gallon of water. A cool green pleasure, this chore—to lie on my belly on the cleft-cedar footbridge with devil's club and old growth overhead, wild ginger, inside-out flower, and violets all around, ferns and moss buffering the brook."

Saturday, April 17, 2010

Homeless and Hopeless in Hermann Park

Houston Texas has a huge homeless population. Not surprising since it's the 4th largest city in the US, and it's blessed with being in a very mild climate.

You see them everywhere, if you pay attention.

Under overpasses, cardboard walls crumple in on meager possessions that only look like refuse to most of the rest of us.

Tucked into empty lots, backed into doorways, people lost from within and invisible from without while away the days that all must run together in a never-ending procession of nightmare and surprise.

We noticed the Houston Homeless on our very first trip there. Those first years' pilgrimages to the cancer hospital included our little dog, who would go to doggy daycare while we were otherwise occupied, and doggy daycare was past the hospitals, past Hermann Park, and just past the Museum District.

That first morning, we were stopped at a stoplight in front of a church. Not Sunday morning, yet the entire yard was filled with a queue of humanity silently awaiting entrance. It's a soup kitchen.

Where the Homeless go during the day I'm not sure, but one winter evening we were retrieving our little dog just after dark, and though the parents and children, bikers and joggers had long left Hermann Park, the Homeless had appeared like Ghost Moths, hovering lightly and almost luminously in their nocturnal perches.

I was so preoccupied with my husband's health; I didn't give much thought to the Homeless of Hermann Park till we were faced with an Incident.

Illness has taken a great financial toll on our family. We no longer have a credit card, and we have very little cash. I try to bring as much extra cash as I can, "just in case," and this particular trip I had brought seven days' worth of cash for what was supposed to be a four day trip. My husband contracted MRSA in hospital and we were there ten days. Not four. Not seven. Ten.

Now, the hospital allows patients to cash one personal check a day, for up to $50.

Our hotel room was $65 per day.

I was able to cobble together enough to survive, stay in the hotel, eat, and coast home on gas fumes, but that little episode gave me pause, and I couldn't help but wonder...

How many of the Hermann Park Homeless have family members in one of the many hospitals of the Hospital District? We came perilously close to "camping" in our auto those last few nights. What if I'd been OUT out of money, not just ALMOST out of money? What if my husband had been delayed by MONTHS instead of days?

In the last eight years we've been with insurance, without insurance, and on Medicare. Ward's been employed and unemployed. We've had medical trips when we've had money and medical trips when I've literally gone begging for funds.

But the one thing that's been lurking at the back of my mind—behind the weedy shrubberies and crouched next to an old shopping cart—is the knowledge that, like so many people who are "one paycheck away from eviction," without our safety net of family and friends, we'd be truly and honestly one medical procedure away from living in Hermann Park.

What happens when the money runs out before the medical emergency is fixed? We're currently here two weeks, with no foreseeable date to go home—ground to a halt by a snowballing hairball of unexpected complications. We thought we'd be here five days—seven at the most. We've got options, and support, and more love than a family can absorb without overflowing, and we're OK. We can weather this storm under roof and with full tummies.

But what if we didn't have those options, support, and love?

What if we didn't have a computer that linked us with people around the world who care about us? What if I'd been working several jobs to keep ahead of disaster while caring for a family and ill husband and didn't have the time, energy, or heart to make and keep friends who we could fall back on?

What if we were truly alone, as so many families are in our fragmented society?

I refuse to leave Ward here, trapped, helpless, and afraid, in a hospital bed. If I had to, I'd live on a park bench to be with him every day.

How many of the Hermann Park Homeless are doing just that? Is that why they seem to disappear during the day? Are they next to the bed of a loved one, holding a hand, reassuring them that everything is all right although it's anything but?

The Hospital District in Houston is the largest in the WORLD—just this cluster of hospitals employs 65,000 people. Every one of those hundred or so waiting in the soup line could slip into any one of those great maws of medical care and be totally not noticed in the crowds.

And how many have left the hospital for the last time, mechanically leaving the empty shell of the worn-out patient, and going through the motions of walking, navigating hallways and crosswalks on automatic pilot, their bodies weighted to the earth while their sanity frantically flutters after the soul of the one just lost—up, up and gone—not caring what happens now to their own broken-hearted shell?

I wonder about these things.

But I'm mortally afraid to know the truth.

17 April 2010 at 11:18pm

Today—more of the same.

They back off of his sedation just a wee bit, and then have to give blood pressure meds and nitroglycerin till he settles down. Repeat.

He'll be quiet, then his legs/arms twitch and he breathes heavily and chews on his tube (they've got a stopper for that) and scrunches up his face in a frown. When he does that, I stop reading, stand up, stroke his forehead, and tell him he's OK, that they are just waking him up really slowly to be sure the graft is safe—always aware that he won't even remember going BACK into surgery, and once he can think straight his first thought will be, "WHAT THE HELL????" and he'll fight like a Big Dog.

So I tell him to try to be calm, to try to concentrate on my hand in his, and the words of the book, which are all wonderfully descriptive and do an excellent job of pulling the reader/listener into the quiet, peaceful wilderness of the Dark Divide of southwestern Washington State.

Twice this afternoon, once when I first arrived and stroked his forehead and told him I was there, and once when I told him I had to leave to get Alec, his face crumpled up and a single tear squeezed out of his closed eye.

Absolutely. Completely. Broke my entire heart.

18 April 2010 at 6:09pm

They said that Ward's not much improved, since they're going so slowly, and he had a few episodes of atrial fib last night (heart tantrums) so had to be medicated each time, but he's not any worse, which in his case, is stellar news.

They changed his sedation to Versed from Propofol (yes—Michael Jackson's drug-o-choice) and he looks more like he's sleeping and less like he's medically paralyzed.

I only stayed two hours today. Alec was alone in the hotel room and I'm uncomfortable leaving him untended for more than just a few hours.

The highlight of my day—my older son called me JUST TO TALK—to see how Ward's doing, how we're doing, and he talked to Alec a good long time too.

THANK YOU, DAVE. YOU'RE A VERY GOOD BOY. ♥

It's only 5pm, but the bed is calling me...

Monday, April 19, 2010

Giving Up the Illusion of Control

I'm an ornery ol' cuss.

Oh, I know on the outside I look pretty harmless—a half-century-old hippie chick with long graying hair, smile lines around my bi-focaled eyes, and gravity obviously luring my "pointier parts" back into Mother Earth. My wardrobe's from Goodwill, I am loathe to wear anything but flip flops, I spend no money on makeup, manicures, or haircuts, and wear only a few cherished but simple pieces of jewelry.

Not a very formidable front.

But on the inside, I've always held that Sicilian Mama belief that most things in the world flat can't run without me at the helm. No one can cook like I can. No one can clean the house like I can. No one can pay the bills, organize our son's schooling, run my place of employment, and the home farm like I can.

Without me supervising, my entire family would be wandering around outside, unfed, unbathed, and probably pants-less.

If anyone offers to help with any of the above, my answer has always been, "No thanks- I'll take care of it."

And I did, for a very long time.

And I still do, mostly.

But something happened about four years ago. My husband's health needs made it impossible for merely me to take care of everything. We were required to spend large amounts of time away from home, and that took me away from the helm, the rudder, the gist of the matters, and left me relying on...other people.

This rankled. A lot. For I still thought I could handle everything alone.

But much as I wanted to, there was no way to feed and care for the farm while I was 200 miles away from it. Friends and neighbors stepped in, and even though they did not do everything exactly as I did, nothing died. In fact, a few things they did differently were so sensible; I smacked myself upside the head in wonder that I'd been doing them otherwise for years.

And much as I wanted to, there was no way to be at my place of employment at the same time I was at the hospital with my husband. So I learned to delegate, and found that my employees were not only willing but also happy to help out and take on additional duties for the duration. And the business did not go to hell in a hand basket.

And even when we ARE home, I've learned that my family consists of intelligent, innovative humans who have both complex thought processes AND opposable thumbs, and that they are capable of helping out on the home front.

The boys cooking dinner with the help of Mrs. Stouffer's every so often will not kill us.

Boys who dust AROUND knick-knacks instead of lifting them and dusting under them do not cause a rift in the time-space continuum.

My husband can, and does, teach our son with a patience and imagination I could never achieve.

They can even (mostly) remember to wear pants outside of the house.

The most difficult thing of all had to do with money.

A lot of our friends and family live far away and cannot come to give actual, physical, haul-the-hay, collect-the-eggs, scrub-the-toilets help. But they want so badly to ease our pain, our hurt, and our difficulties that they send their love in the form of cash.

This bothered me more than anything else, this sending of money. It smacked of neediness, of helplessness, of weakness.

So I'd refuse politely but firmly, sending money back to the gifter while simultaneously worrying about how to pay for the next medical disaster.

Until.

One of my friends lost patience with my bullheadedness.

She railed at me in frustration, demanding me to put myself in their shoes, to reverse the roles. "What would YOU do? If any one of us needed anything you'd be there to help in a heartbeat, and if you couldn't come personally, YOU'D SEND MONEY and be offended if it were returned".

She told me that by not allowing my friends to help us, I was doing THEM a great dis-service, denying them the only option open to them to ease my family's distress, our worry, our hardship.

I learned to say "thank you" graciously and sincerely.

When asked what we need, I've learned to answer honestly with our current concerns instead of saying, "Nothing, we're fine," when we so clearly are not.

Oh, don't get me wrong. I'm still a nit-picky eagle-eyed terror on medical staff and am daily an unreasonable harpy to my family.

But I've learned now that I don't have to shoulder the entire load the entire time the entire way—that the only one who even expected that of me was...me.

19 April 2010 at 8:27pm

Ward's poor throat grew two kinds of staph and he's now got pneumonia, so they're hitting him with different/more antibiotics. He's so thin now (and he didn't have any meat to spare) that his ribs are setting several inches above his tummy and defined like a skeleton.

I was going to make a 24-hour run home (the ten hours of driving INclusive) tomorrow, but have decided to wait till later next week. He should be (please please please) awake and in a regular room by then. (I almost added "and out of the woods" but caught myself. Considering the last two weeks, there will be no "out of the woods" talk till we're literally back IN OUR WOODS.)

He's still not awake or very responsive; although, when I got there and took his hand, it was very still, with just tiny faint random twitches.

We've always had a code for when we're holding hands--three squeezes "I. Love. You." So I deliberately squeezed three times.

Pause.

Then still faint, and not quite a squeeze, but more than a twitch and very distinct—1-2-3.

19 April 2010 at 9:09pm

Well, he's not opened his eye yet, so I've got precious little to go on as far as anything but very brief flashes of Who-ville "I am here I am here I am here" communication.

The ICU nurses seem very good, and the ICU doctor seems excellent. When I come in, I can tell he's been cared for, kept clean, and there are pillows/cushions in thoughtful places to take pressure from the various boxes and tubings lying all over/in/around him.

Thrush is actually what they were looking for when they found the staph.

Our friend, whose son was recently in a motorcycle accident and then a coma for sixteen days, said Philip remembers nothing of the sixteen days he was "out", but just in case, I keep telling Ward:

-You are OK.
-They are just waking you up REALLY slowly for the safety of your graft.
-You are OK.
-I'm right here, and if I'm not right in the room with you, I'm just two miles from here at the hotel with Alec, and we're waiting for you.
-You are OK.

20 April 2010 at 9:37pm

Ward's heart is behaving, but he's now running fever. They scoped his lung through his breathing tube (so, as non-invasively as possible) and vacuumed out his left lung, removing (TMI warning for the faint-of-heart) almost a pint of pus.

While they did "the procedure," I went in search of Patient
Advocacy, thus far elusive this whole last week—I'd call up there
and get their voicemail 100% of the time. I found their offices
tucked in a corner behind a small sign, walked in, and asked to see
a real person. The girl was flummoxed as to who to have me talk to
since each department has their own advocate assigned and he's
now being treated by SEVEN different departments (ICU, cardio,
head/neck, pain management, reconstructive surgery, internal
medicine, psychiatric).

Finally I had to get back to Ward to talk to the doctor after the
procedure and I told her, "I want a real person, in ICU, before 5pm
or tomorrow, I will by god find whoever I go to to complain about
the people you are supposed to go to to complain."

Ten minutes later there was a Patient Advocate in ICU looking for
me.

He asked how he could help and I told him we needed a place to sit
down and he needed to take notes. I told him the ENtire story of
our last fifteen (!?) days. I told him I don't have a complaint about
any individual—everyone seems competent, sincere and caring—
but that parts of the system clearly suck and need addressed.

I told him Ward needs glasses before he wakes up and he agreed.
I'm to get his script from the eyeglass place in Tyler and he'll have
some made NOW. They are also replacing the books that were
lost.

So we'll see, but I'm cautiously optimistic that this guy will, yanno,
advocate for us.

They are still trying to slowly wake Ward up, hoping to remove the
tube in the next 48 hours or so.

When I got there, his eye was open, but not focusing on anything. I
got no hand squeezes or twitches today.

By the time I left, his pupil was sliding over in my direction and I asked him, "Honey, do you see me?" He nodded faintly.

I asked him, "Honey, am I a meerkat?" He frowned and shook his head imperceptibly.

So far so good.

I told him when I left that he needs to fight like hell from the inside and I'll fight like hell from the outside and we'll meet in the middle. He sighed and the smile lines showed at the corner of his eye.

21 April 2010 at 9:03pm

Hey—guess who I saw today?

Ward. Ward Dixon.

Ya'll might remember him...

I walked into his room and there he was—no breathing tube, eye open, happy to see me.

Now, a quick assessment still shows stitches on his head, neck, and leg, the 'detour' tube up one nostril and a feeding tube up the other, a pik line into an artery on his right arm for ease of blood draws for labs and three (I think) IV's in his left arm, EKG heart monitor stickers all over, a drain tube in his leg for that graft donor area, pressure socks/shoelets on his feet and a ... "personal territory" catheter.

BUT

Under all that is Ward.

His fever's down and he knows who I am and is able to answer questions readily, though not easily since his throat still hurts a lot and he's really, really dry.

He said, "OK, let's go."

I said, "What do you mean, dear?"

He said, "Help me get up and let's go."

I tried telling him how long he'd been "down" and the nurse verified that.

He said, "Shhh," and tried to get up.

I said, "You're too weak, dear—you have to be awake awhile before they let you get up."

And he said, "Shhh," and tried to get up.

Ten days I wait for him to talk to me, and in five minutes he dismissed me twice.

So the nurse rearranged him on the bed and sat him up some and I asked him:

-Did he remember going in for the first surgery? "Yes"
-Did he remember the little medication problems? "They poisoned me". I told him yes, yes they did, twice, but they won't do that again.
-Did he remember I'd been sick? "Yes."
-Did he remember going in for the second surgery? "Yes."
-Did he know I'd been there all afternoon every afternoon? "Yes."
-Did he remember me reading to him? "Yes."
-Did he enjoy the book? "Yes."
-Did he want me to read to him today? "No."

He wanted conversation today, even if it was interspersed with pleas to help him up and out of there that were summarily denied.

At 6pm I said I needed to leave—visiting hours were over and I had to get back to the hotel to Alec and he said, "Yes, I know that."

I got a kiss and an "I love you" and I left him listening to Animal Planet on the TV.

Alec and I grilled little skillet steaks on the hotel grill, I nuke-baked some potatoes and steamed some broccoli, and Alec proclaimed it AWESOME (of course, I let him be the Grill master—playing with fire is always awesome).

An early evening here tonight.

If I show up tomorrow and they've made him worse (again), I'll really have to hurt someone.

22 April 2010 at 12:57am

Well, shit. That lasted what? Six hours?

So I called up there, anticipating Alec could, yanno, TALK to his dad for the first time in ten days and the nurse said, "He's sleeping."

Really

Further questioning revealed that he WAS calm and easy-going after I left, then they decided to suction out more of the yack that's still coming out of his throat and lung.

He didn't like that.

He's now not letting anyone near him and I assume he is tied back to the bed.

She said she knew his throat is probably a little sore" after being intubated for surgery, but they had to suction and the orders were for as little (preferably no more) sedation. That she just gave IV pain meds (NOT Dilaudid—at least they didn't do THAT) and now he's resting.

Oh, baby. That was MY last straw.

Really? Really? Was she aware of just HOW sore his mouth and throat are??? That he had surgery FIFTEEN days ago and was intubated, then suffered insanity for a week while complaining of a pain threshold NINE sore throat that they never swabbed so most likely when they did the SECOND surgery TEN DAYS ago they probably stuffed all that crap directly into his lung and that he's now been intubated TEN DAYS- **THAT THAT'S HOW SORE HIS THROAT IS???**

Did they think to use something topical first so it wouldn't hurt, or LORD ABOVE GIVE THE PAIN MEDICATION *BEFORE* HURTING HIM???

Ya. No. They didn't.

She said, "Well, the other nurse did say he's better when you're here."

I said, "Of COURSE he's better when I'm there—whenever I leave ya'll HURT HIM. Do NOT—NOT—hurt him anymore tonight. If you must suction again, I understand that, but either give pain meds first and give them time to work, or get the DOCTOR in there to sedate him a bit, because right this minute, I have completely, totally HAD IT with that hospital."

She said she understood, and repeated that he's "sleeping." No, he's not. He's staying still so they leave him the hell alone.

When I left tonight, he was lucid and understood where I was going and why. I set him up with the TV clicker and asked if he was ok.

He said, "I'm afraid. I'm afraid."

I'm headed to bed. I've got heads to roll tomorrow.

22 April 2010 at 11:34pm

Ward's about the same today. He can whisper a few words, and nod yes or shake his head no—enough for his wife to know exactly what he means, which is something the staff is now very, very aware of.

Physical therapy came before I got there and had him sit up in the bed with his feet over the edge for the first time. They said, "He didn't want to do it." When the diabetes lady came to check his feet, she found under his pressure socks that he's got terrible gout in both feet and ankles. Gee—I wonder why he didn't appreciate having his legs hauled around and dangled over the edge of the bed??? So they've restarted him on his gout meds.

I talked to both the patient advocate and the surgeon about how this inpatient trip has taken a good, trusting, calm patient and turned him into a paranoid crab-ass, and it ain't the drugs anymore—it's completely justified.

They both agreed.

That he's now mortally, truly afraid to be there alone is not good for his healing or the mental peace of his family.

They've both talked to the staff in ICU, and we will all be talking to the charge nurse once he's back on the 11th floor for, in the

surgeon's words, "A little staff re-education." The surgeon told me
we are not the first of his families who've had a "sub-optimal
experience" (how's that for hospital administration jargon?).

The patient advocate has in hand both the prescription and the
frame style to get his glasses done and will be replacing the books
once I get him the titles/authors.

I was there when the respiratory therapist did the suctioning this
morning, and directed her to give IV pain meds FIRST, and then
wait 10 minutes. I told her, "While you're waiting, go get some
numbing gel"—and she did. I held his hand while she suctioned,
and afterwards I asked him if that was better than last night. He
nodded emphatically. The RT wrote on his chart how to suction
from now on.

The day nurse had him yesterday and is very good. She instructed
the night nurse to do NOTHING to hurt him, and the daytime RT
is giving oral directions as well to the nighttime RT for suctioning.

I just talked to him and asked if anyone has hurt him since I left.
He whispered, "No." I told him I'm at the hotel. "OK." That I'll be
up after lunch. "OK." Told him goodnight and I love you. "I love
you too"—twice.

Absolute. Music. Absolutely.

...Speaking of hospital administration, Hospital Administrator Dr.
Mendelsohn's office is apparently not IN the hospital. *How
Convenient.*

Of course, that's merely a challenge to be overcome, and I loves
me a challenge.

Oh yeah—
Alec had a date today. The 23-year-old absolutely gorgeous
daughter of the kids' room lady snatched Alec for the afternoon.
They went paddle boating and out to lunch at Chili's, WHICH
ALEC PAID FOR.

Afterwards I said, "She sure is pretty," and he looked at me with his best "Girls are Gross" 10-year-old look, then shrugged and sorta smiled and said, "Yep. She sure is."

23 April 2010 at 7:45pm

When I got to Ward's room today, the physical therapist had him sitting up in bed with his legs over the side. He's very weak, and sorta keeps tipping over, and there's no strength at all in his arms, but hey—he was sitting up and making sensible, if still whispered, conversation.

He's still pretty fuzzyheaded. We'd be talking about Alec and Joe, and he'd be asking and answering right on target, then he asked how Murdie is—his mom, who passed on eight years ago. I told him she's fine.

Then he wanted to know when we can go home. Can we go tonight? I said no. Tomorrow? I said, "I'm sorry, dear—your brain may be ready to go home, but your body needs to do a lot of catching up." I assured him that Alec and I are here till he's ready, and then we'll all go home.

He said, "OK. So. Do we live in an apartment or something?"

I said, "No, dear—we've got a big ol' house in the country with turkeys on the porch and chickens in the yard" and he said, "Wow. That sounds wonderful."

So, maybe his brain needs to catch up a little too...

They are tentatively talking about moving him to the regular floor tomorrow or the next day, although he needs a lot of physical building up (he's down to 160, so he lost another almost 20 pounds since surgery), and obviously there are still cobwebs in his head. So still a long way from discharge, poor baby, but he's calm and lovable and there's even a twinkle of humor there.

I was explaining to the doctor that agitation in him is NOT normal. That if he complains it's because whatever they are doing HURTS and to STOP. That he's the patient, kind, gentle half of our marriage, and I'm the pointy, irritable, excitable one.

Whisper from the bed:

"Boy, THAT'S the damn truth."

...Golly, I've missed him.

Alec left with Dorothy from the kids' room, and her family. They're off to eat pizza and play games till they drop. They said they'll have him back to the hotel by 11, but don't wait up...

I'm here at the hotel catching a bite to eat, then will go back up to see Ward for the 8-10pm visiting hours. I missed a lot of the afternoon ones trying to contact Dr. Mendelsohn, President of MDA. I got as far as his secretary on the phone and she assured me that, although Dr. Mendelsohn isn't available to speak, she'd have someone in "the Executive Branch" call me back. What I got was the Patient Advocacy Supervisor, who seemed miffed that I'd go "over her head."

She ain't seen nuthin' yet—just wait till Monday...

23 April 2010 at 7:51pm

I drafted the following missive, which has been delivered to the GOOD patient advocate, Farhad, and he's getting a copy to everyone involved, including Dr. Mendelsohn:

Notes on MDAnderson—the Good, the Bad, and the Frustrating
4/23/2010

Outstanding people at MDA-

Dr. Hanasono- Reconstructive surgery
Dr. Adelman- Reconstructive surgery
Katie DeLuccia- Reconstructive surgery PA
Dorothy- the kids' room lady
Martha Ashenbrenner
Farhad Tehrani
Cora and Maria on the 11th floor

Issues and Examples

Continuity of record/test results/ history between shifts and doctors

-An order for Tylenol administration was given when blood work less than 7 days prior shows beginning liver disease.
-The re-admission of Dilaudid after doctors' orders to discontinue because of a (now known) violent allergy should never have happened. Ever.
-Having to repeat history verbally over and over and over again—not recent updates; full history—is exhausting to the family and very unprofessional.
-Doctors are not checking most recent labwork/tests/xrays before giving new prognoses and plans.
-There's no overlap in care. Entire caregiver group changes out every 12 hours.

Balancing protocol and the smooth running of a hospital with compassion and common sense

-The across-the-board refusal of floor staff to respect an open communication request for a non-lucid patient is frustrating and shows lack of compassion.

-Subjecting a patient to uncomfortable procedures needlessly is cruel and unnecessary.

-Losing personal items integral to a patient's well-being—prescription eyeglasses and reading material—is sloppy management.

-Neglecting to get a simple throat swab on a patient complaining of 'threshold 9' pain sore throat is basic lack of care.

Accessibility to Patient Advocacy

Patient Advocates need to be available to answer calls at time of first contact—it's not comforting to get voice mail 100% of the time and play phone tag for over a week.

Concerns and Suggestions

Due to an accumulation of all the above scenarios, you now have a patient who is mortally afraid of being left alone in your hospital, something he's never been before. This makes it very difficult for him to do the hard work of healing, and very difficult for his family to have a moments' peace unless we're watching over him. Such an atmosphere should not be in any medical facility, much less one of this caliber.

While we understand that the Human Condition comes with ups and downs, it's very, very discouraging for me, as the spouse of a patient, to spend hours with him, and when I leave he's better mentally and when I return he's much worse—not just because of his medical condition or drugged mindset—but because of something the staff is directly doing to him or not doing for him.

In a state-of-the-art hospital, it's inconceivable to me how archaic the record keeping is—and actually a testament to the staff that they are able to care for patients at all considering the cumbersome nightmares laughingly defined as "patient charts." You have the money and the facility—why is it so hard to move beyond doctors' hand scrawled directives buried quickly in a ream of paper?

To stagger who changes each shift would go a long way to giving patients a feeling of security and staff a feeling of competence. I no longer give any credence to being told, "He's resting," or "He's doing better," if there has been a shift change since my last check, because I've found in reality, neither is the case—that as long as he's not screaming or causing any trouble, he's "resting and better."

Every employee needs to remember at all times that they have in their care fathers, mothers, children—not just "Bed #34." Each patient is a person, not just a body to be tended. That it's not only the doctors who are sworn to "First—do no harm," but every single nurse, aide, technician and staff member.

While I appreciate the chance to have a conference with floor staff regarding my husband's care, it's heartbreaking that such a thing even needs to be brought up.

My husband has a lot of health issues, but that is (I think) more common than not at this hospital. People come here BECAUSE their local hospitals cannot care for the scope of difficulty these patients are faced with. It's frightening to me to consider the many, many people who do NOT speak up. If they go home well, small frustrations are forgotten, and if they don't go home at all, those frustrations become obsolete.

I sincerely hope that this list does not need additions in the time we have left at MDAnderson, and fervently hope that our experience from here on out is positive, and that when we need to seek medical attention again, we'll be comfortable returning to your hospital, and not feel we'll be better served taking our chances at our tiny local hospital or an alternative medicine center—both of which look pretty good to us right now.

Respectfully,

Sheri Dixon
Patient Ward Dixon #******

Friday, April 23, 2010

Fish Out Of Water Desires Rental Lungs and Feet

I'm a Leo.

The feline fire sign.

But I'm not an inside cat by any stretch of the imagination. I prefer outside to indoors unless it's below about 50 degrees—then you'll find me curled up by the fireplace. I'm a fire sign. I crave warmth.

Even wildly mis-planted in Wisconsin for my first 35 years, my preference was always to be outside as long as the above temperature requirement was met, and even then, during the long winters (which last from October 1st thru May up yonder) I'd make a break for the outdoor world frantically every month or so when a flash of Nature would lure me out into it and I'd breathe deeply, the icy air filling my dusty lungs. I can't take a full breath inside.

There are eight hours or so every fall that hold the perfect autumn hues in a grasp of perfection. Not the sunny, blue-skied days of magazine layouts, but one day with heavy charcoal clouds pressing down on the woods and the lowering sun infusing and drenching each leaf with glowing vibrancy—denying the reality of the next days' withering, browning, brittle descent into quietly composting anonymity.

The aftermath of a midnight snow storm—the full moon seemingly within reach, and so brilliant the stars fall out of the sky and lie twinkling at your feet, each snowflake reflecting a faraway sun in the deep of an earthly night.

Early spring, when the rain falls before the air is warm, encasing everything in a transparent glistening frozen cocoon—tree, twig, budding leaf and flower—all surprised and often broken by the very substance they need to live finally come after a long winter, but just that much too soon. Timing is everything.

So even in Wisconsin, (Native American for "Land of the Three Day Summer") my natural environment was Outside.

I preferred camping to shopping, hiking to TV watching, a day at the out-of-the-way nature preserve to the stuffifying interior of the school building.

Even as a grown-up, gainful employment needed, if not actual exposure to Outside, at the very least to be where I could see it—to know if it were morning or evening by the sky instead of the timeclock, if it were sunny or raining by sight and not the weather channel.

Working for a flower shop as an all-around gal, I was out delivering arrangements one day and one bright bouquet went to a medical transcription office (in the days before home computers, that's what they did). I walked into the windowless, music-free office filled wall to wall with women wearing headsets and concentrating on their work. The only sound was the ticking of keys. I felt panicked, strangled, it was suddenly very difficult to breathe as I realized that this was their life—eight hours a day, five days a week—and I thought:

"This is hell."

Finally unable to ignore that little voice screaming "MIGRATE SOUTH" any longer, I found what I was looking for—East Texas, filled with forests, water, hills, and the lazy luxury of tremendously long wildflower-filled springs and crazy quilt colored autumns with just a smidgen of "wow—hot" or "kinda chilly" dividing them.

Now my Outside Spirit is in its element. Even when inside, our windows are generally wide open, our house merely a roof and a few walls giving the illusion of shelter, and even when too cold, it's not deadly frostbite cold, just mildly annoying for a few days.

Except.

These last few years have seen many times that I've been forced Inside. More than just inside an office building or behind a desk, I've been bent, folded, spindled, and crammed into the very un-natural element of a very large city.

Now, I honestly can't say I've hated every minute of it.

I've hated the REASON we're here—just one of a huge herd of Cancer Families making weary frightened pilgrimages to lay our loved ones on the altar of medicine, leaving sacrificial parts and pieces behind.

But as granola munchin' tree huggin' nature lovin' as I am, I've always appreciated the things only large urban areas can offer— museums, theater, music, culture both high falutin' and local—and have always thoroughly enjoyed my excursions into large metropolitan areas from Chicago to Miami, from Los Angeles to Washington DC.

My terms, my choice, my call as to when to escape back to the quiet and peace of the forest, cherishing and grateful for what I've been able to experience in the urban jungle, and so thankful I don't have to live there.

We're currently on our 18th day of a six-day trip to Houston.

My husband lays in ICU, the very epitome of "ravaged and wasted" after a string of events only the devil himself could put so cleverly together. He's fighting for life, for his wife, for his son—

and, in tiny steps, is climbing out inch by torturous inch back to his family.

And while I feel enormous guilt at every moment not spent at his side, I also know that I need to be "out here" for his son, that both our son and I need something other than the suffocating surroundings of the hospital, that even while our hearts break at the knowledge that Ward's trapped there, in that bed, inside his faltering body, we know that when he wakes fully up he'll not be angry about the hours we spent away from his bedside, but all those we did.

So we go. And do. And see. And every experience we try to engrave on our memories to share with him, make plans to do again, with him.

Being an Outside animal trapped in an Inside world, I can only tolerate the hospital for a few hours at a time. Then I must flee, literally, if only for 10 minutes, and I stop at the cafe for something to drink or a snack and maneuver through the interior maze, out the door, between cars and buses and taxicabs and ambulances to the tiny garden planted artfully and hopefully betwixt the hospital and the busy street. And I sit, face lifted towards the sun, shoes kicked off, eyes closed, breathing slowly if not deeply for the smog and the exhaust fumes. Before heading back inside, I bury my nose for one deep breath stolen from the heart of a rose—not my favorite flower, but as close to heaven as I can get right here, right now.

My family has been forced to adapt to this environment, and while gleaning and benefiting from the many offerings afforded by it, we are not thriving.

We all three of us look to the day we can turn in our rented lungs and feet and dive joyfully (if exhausted) back into our beloved Pineywoods, leaving only a slight and quickly fading ripple on the surface of Houston. To a time when we will again only emerge by choice, and not be forced out by circumstance.

23 April 2010 at 11:16pm

Yea Verily, and on the Twelfth Day he was moved from ICU back onto the 11th floor, where he was given into the kind mercies of the three nurses who were most helpful during his last stay.

And Lo, tho 'twas late, the Charge Nurse herself came and introduced herself to his wife, assuring her of the wisdom of trusting the staff of the 11th floor, where it was vowed he would have a peaceful stay till his strength returns and he is discharged from their care.

Amen.

Ha. Think my letter has already made the rounds?

24 April 2010 at 1:36pm

When they told us in ICU they thought he'd recover better up on the floor, I asked point blank, "Why? That's where most of the stuff to make him worse went on—the extra Dilaudid, the not letting him call me, the not swabbing his throat, the losing of his stuff..."

Did they understand why I wasn't breathing a sigh of relief that he was going right back up there???

They did, I think, and relayed it before we got there.

We're headed up there in a little bit, and there are clear skies over Houston, so any thunder you may hear from this direction will tell the tale...

And I don't care how exemplary his care is from here on out—that I needed to go to ANY length to get "special treatment" is sorry, plain and simple.

24 April 2010 at 10:24pm

So far so good as far as care—at 3pm, Miss Alicia, the "sitter" Ward liked best, showed up to sit with him. He's not fractious, or irritable, or paranoid, and he's so weak he couldn't get up the momentum to fall out of bed (truth), so I asked why she was assigned to him.

She said, "Well, they did call me in special. I'm supposed to be on vacation, but I like Mr. Dixon, so I came."

Really.

Interesting.

So we met the daytime nurse, who was very nice, and the nighttime nurse, also very sweet. We told especially the night nurse that if he wants to call the hotel to let him, and she agreed.

Unfortunately, I don't think that's going to happen tonight since he only knows who I am about half the time yet. He's still so very fuzzy he can't answer questions about our home, or life, or his brothers, and he called me by his ex-wife's name once (I'll smack him for that once he's 100%), but he knows his boy every time and without fail.

So, baby steps. We'll take it.

Alec has been asking to "do something downtown," so when Ward fell asleep after Miss Alicia got there, we took the metro-rail downtown ($2.50—an excellent value) to the International Festival. Alec said he was hankerin' after some jambalaya.

After sitting down a minute (the metro-rail makes me woozy) we walked to the festival, paid to get in ($17), found the food, realized we needed coupons, not money, found the coupon tent, bought coupons, got a lemonade and the jambalaya ($10), which Alec looked sorta funny at, but he ate it and proclaimed it "good."

He also got to try out some congas, which was totally awesome.

Then we walked back to the metro, rode back to the hospital, and on the way up to Ward's room Alec said, "Yanno, I thought jambalaya was more like soup".

Apparently the food he was hankering for was GUMBO.

I'll kill him later. I'm pooped.

25 April 2010 at 7:48pm

They found his glasses and books on the far side of the floor, in someone's office, in a bag with his name/patient number on it. Even though he's not strong enough yet to even hold a small book (really), at least he can watch TV now—he's been missing basketball.

Today Ward told me that most of the stuff coming out of his mouth doesn't make a damn bit of sense. And then he chuckled and shook his head like he was trying to clear cobwebs.

We got him into a wheelchair and Alec drove him around the floor a few times, then he sat in a regular chair for about 30 minutes—he still can't stand on his own and sorta flops forward in the chair.

He would seem to understand something, and then two seconds later completely contradict himself.

I didn't ask directly if he knew who I was, but he kept calling me "baby," and told the nurse that I'm "such a damn hard-head" when I wouldn't help get him up and get dressed to go with us when we left, so I'm guessing he knew.

I have to keep reminding him that he's been very, very sick, and needs to be patient and let his body heal. He'll agree, and then say, "OK- help me up- let's go."

When we left, the nurse was talking him out of following us...

26 April 2010 at 11:32pm

Is Ward better physically? A little bit. He can sit up by himself, but not stand on his own yet, and even though they haven't removed his feeding tube, they are allowing him anything he wants to drink—CAUTIOUSLY, with supervision. He chose and enjoyed several sips of ginger ale—the first thing he's had to drink in three weeks.

Is Ward better mentally? Yes and no. When I got there today, he smiled and called me Angel Pumpkin and his little Boxfish (Ya— we're a creepy old mushy mushy couple), but continued to be easily frustrated and agitated.

Here's what I figured out. If he wants to do something he's not allowed to do, like get dressed and leave the hospital (which he insists on doing every five minutes or so), saying, "No dear, you can't do that yet," even if followed by a rational calm explanation, gets scowling and cursing. Saying, "Yes dear, we'll do that as soon as..." and the exact same rational calm explanation will elicit a sigh of acceptance...for about five minutes, when it starts over again.

We watched *Land of the Lost* with Will Ferrell, and he laughed at all the right parts, was happy to see Alec when I retrieved him from work at doggy daycare (although he doesn't remember doggy daycare at all and the whole, "Alec is working at doggy daycare" thing sorta went over his head) and seemed content to stay with tonight's sitter, Myrna, although he said, "See you in a little bit" in response to our, "See you tomorrow."

Baby steps.

27 April 2010 at 1:10am

Alec brought a little photo album with pictures of himself at one of the tae kwon do tournaments, and on his bike, and with and a bunch of our farm and critters to show the kids' room lady. He's given it to his dad for the duration to help him remember…home.

He's a very good boy.

27 April 2010 at 9:44pm

So, today—a lot better physically. Ward's walking a few steps at a time with a walker and sitting in the chair longer. I also got him to eat a few spoonfuls of soup and yogurt. He's so "under-conditioned" (nice medical term, ain't it?) that they won't remove the feeding tube till he's able to feed himself everything he needs to progress.

Mentally, he's still pretty fuzzy. Can't answer questions about our home and life, but is in generally good spirits and pleasant to those around him.

Unfortunately, he's starting to remember the recent past.

Specifically, his SECOND SURGERY, which he told me about step-by-step, through tears, right before we left. Every step, from being intubated, to the pre-surgical scrubbing and shaving, to the cutting, to trying frantically to wake up and being pushed back down over and over again (when he was having his heart failure?).

There's no way he would know each step and what it involved, but they were right on target—and if I find out that one of the surgical team is named Jerry, I think I'll lose MY mind.

He said, "They tried to kill me. I didn't want to die, but they kept trying to kill me."

He asked me, "Why would they do that? How could they do something so cruel? I know I'm just a broken down old man, but that's no reason to be so heartless."

Shit. No wonder his brain has taken a vacation...

28 April 2010 at 9:46am

We were supposed to be gone a week. Ten days at most. I cleverly pre-paid every bill both at home and at work. Unfortunately, we've been gone almost a month and they're all due again. I HAVE to go home and tend to our bills and the work bills.

I can do this. We can visit Ward this morning, drive home (five hours), take care of everything, sleep for a few hours, get up, drive back (five hours), and be back in the hospital room by lunchtime tomorrow. So I'm...

...Packing the car, going to see Ward, and then driving home.

I don't wanna leave Ward, even for 30 hours...

Depending on his "fuzzy factor," I'll probably tell him something along the lines of "we have to run a bunch of work errands today and get Alec ready to start training with Master Ellis on Friday. Stupid stuff I've been neglecting—it'll take all day. We'll call you in between errands and see you tomorrow."

Close enough, think?

Poor Alec—I cried all the way home. I've never made that drive...without Ward. I had a meltdown at Tractor Supply, flew through work like a madwoman, slept two hours fitfully—it was awful being in our bed...alone—and then drove back to Houston like the Hounds of Hell were nipping at our heels.

29 April 2010 at 9:02pm

Ward.
Is.
Better.

He is steady walking across the room with the walker, but very easily tired.

His voice is stronger, and he recognized most of the photos in the little book today.

He talked about camping on our land and how he hopes we get wood ducks in the nest boxes this year.

He still balks when I tell him he can't leave the hospital just yet—that he needs to be well enough for the feeding tube, drains, IV's and URINARY CATHETER to be removed, but as soon as that's all done, we'll be perfectly a-OK to work on getting his strength back AT HOME.

I didn't talk to any doctors today, so I'll get all the "official updates" tomorrow.

But right now, I feel better.

And yanno, that's what matters.

...Cuz it's all about *me.*

I am a little tired...driving almost 600 miles of "errands" in 24 hours'll do that to ya...

30 April 2010 at 10:21pm

Good news first: they took out the drains, the feeding tube, the catheter, and the stitches. They want to watch him over the weekend before taking out the IV to make sure the pneumonia doesn't boomerang back.

Other good news: I told them I don't want him put into rehab, which is the course of action they want me to do. But I want to take him home and have a home nurse come once a day—and they said since either myself or Joe are always there, we can do that.

Which is awesome since I couldn't see how putting an already fuzzy-headed patient into a totally NEW atmosphere for six weeks (or more) would do anything but set him back.

Bad news is mine, not Ward's. Ya'll ready to post bail when I literally knock two shrinks' heads together?

They came by to assess his progress. I asked them (outside his room and across the floor) if they'd gotten my email about his surgical memory.

They were just short of hostile. Said it was a delusion—explained to me (like I'm five) that if he were struggling and awake they couldn't have done surgery.

Looked at me daring me to contradict their superior intelligence.

Fools.

I told them I know HIM. I've been with him through the delusions and horrors the doctors THERE had put him through, been through post-op fogginess many, many times, and this is different. This IS real. Not consciously real—but on some level he KNEW what they did and FELT what they did. That his attitude before and after telling me was lucid and calm.

I was not accusing anyone of doing something purposely cruel. I was just (apparently stupidly) asking them for suggestions to help him put this MEMORY away—at peace—so he can continue to heal and remember things not horrifying.

They kept saying, "Well, you can't argue with a delusion, but you can't tell him it's real, either." I said, "You have no idea if it's real or not. Don't you dare drug him. Don't go near him again." And I walked away.

Seriously—you can't tell me in a hospital that size that NO ONE has EVER had that same memory.

The one shrink was pretty new and young, and she kept nervously looking at the other one.

I wasn't looking for a fight. I was looking for advice from someone who is supposedly a professional. To be told right out that he can't possibly remember what happened is bullshit. No one has any idea what's in someone else's' mind and if a SHRINK doesn't know that, what the hell?

I respect the doctors who say, "I don't know—lets find out" 1,000 times more than the ones who say, "Because I say so" when that's all they've got to offer because they DON'T KNOW.

To their credit, the surgical team didn't say it's NOT a memory. all they could do was reassure me that during surgery he was not moving, making noise, or fluttering his eyelids—all signs that he would've been "too light."

They were horrified by his memory and so very sorry.

As I said—I never thought they did it on purpose.

But that doesn't make it any less real.

01 May 2010 at 8:23pm

Sort of discouraged today. He was very fuzzy again and didn't understand that "home" is a five hour drive, remembered we were staying at the hotel, but then asked how things are at the theater and to be careful in the hallway (which the hotel doesn't have), and he was easily irritated at anything either Alec or I said.

Alec and I went to the dragon boat races down on the bayou and he was disappointed this morning when we saw him that he couldn't go with us. So we videoed the races on my phone and brought him lunch from the Thai restaurant we ate at—brought the races to HIM—and he was pretty surly and dismissive of it all and us.

I guess it's going to be up and down for quite a while, but the good days just make the bad ones seem worse.

What a whiner, hey?

03 May 2010 at 12:23am

Ward's attitude was good today—mainly quiet and contented, even though he seems more painful again. He's got no meat at all on his bones, so everywhere that touches anything hurts, and he's cold all the time—he's just skin and bones against the world. Just walking the three steps to the bathroom exhausts him, and then he forgets why he's there and what to do about it.

He's still very fuzzy—trying to change the TV channels by pointing the phone at the TV and pressing the numbers, leaving the phone off the hook and then being angry that I didn't call him, not being able to remember anything I tell him for more than five minutes. He'll ask me a question and I'll answer it and he'll ask it again a few minutes later—All. Day. Long. He keeps forgetting he's in the hospital, speaks a fair amount of strange German/Spanish gibberish, and for some reason he's seeing small furry monkeys all over the room.

He's not really eating or drinking enough to sustain a gerbil. Unless he's got a 'sitter' with him, he doesn't eat. He's not of a mind to think to order for himself, and even if asked he'll say, "No, I'm OK, thanks."

So I PUT juice in front of him, which he drank right up, and I went and got him coffee and some apple cake (he did have the sense to say didn't hold a candle to MINE), which he ate right up. I got him a big bowl of fruit, which he ate right up, and I brought him some rotisserie chicken and some homemade mac and cheese and a dinner roll for supper, and he ate a good 1/2 of it.

Tomorrow's goals—to talk to ALL his doctors—surgeon, cardio (I don't even know if anyone has told him he's in heart FAILURE yet), pain management, physical therapy and get a game plan together that everyone agrees on, call the patient advocate and air a few grievances about the psychiatrist, and most importantly, get him into the hospital barber shop. His gorgeous waist-long hair is in a solid mat against his head. Once that's taken care of, I will, by god, get him into the shower for the first time in almost a month.

03 May 2010 at 12:57am

All other hospitals we've been in have given you a menu to choose items from for the next day's meals, which they then deliver to the rooms three times a day. MDA uses a room service type menu— you can order anything, anytime, and they bring it individually—ut that means it's up to the patient and their family to make sure they, yanno, *eat.*

They've been sponge-bathing him. All the sutures and drains just came out the other day, and I understand not wanting to make the matted mane of hair worse by getting it wet without benefit of some serious conditioner/detangler. The barbershop hopefully will be able to save it. He was either insane and not letting anyone near him, or unconscious in ICU for most of the last month—not really good times to "do his hair."

03 May 2010 at 10:16am

Ok. The barber agreed that Ward really can't endure sitting and waiting for a haircut at the barbershop, and that his long hair is most likely a goner—it seriously doesn't look like hair anymore, it's so matted.

Add to that that he's very tender-headed—He goes, "Ow" if I accidentally hit a little snarl when I'm braiding it on the best of days—and I just can't make him put up with trying to salvage it.

Since he's still so fuzzy, I think it'd be easier all around to just start over. It'll be easier to take care of for now, and it grows incredibly fast. So the barber is putting a sterilized clippers and a cape in a bag for me, along with shampoo for after the shearing.

That's this afternoon's little project.

I called up there since I told Ward I'd call him between eight and nine today and he's not answering the phone. It just doesn't occur to him to do so. That tells me he's got no sitter again today.

So I called and talked to his nurse for the day and asked if Ward had had breakfast (I knew the answer, but wanted to see what he said). He said, "He's sipping a little ginger ale."

Ya. That's what *I* brought him LAST NIGHT.

So I told him he needs to go in there and HELP WARD get something to eat NOW.

Is it just me, or is today shaping up to be really, really long???

03 May 2010 at 1:59pm

We have a plan.

I just spent almost an hour on the phone with the surgeon, god bless him.

-They are going to tentatively shoot for a Thursday discharge, mainly because he's confused (like I am) as to why Ward's on two kinds of blood thinners and his levels today show he's maybe a little TOO thin now. A Thursday discharge will give them time to correct anything.

-They'll do a scan if we want them to, to see if he has, in fact, had a stroke, but neither one of us is sure if he's lucid enough to lie still for the 20 minutes it'll take, and our plans on how to proceed won't change either way.

-Other than the blood-thinning issue, physically he just needs building up slowly.

-Mentally, we're going to try taking him home first, and he's going to make sure that if it's too confusing for him, or he becomes a "wanderer" to the point of us not being able to keep up with him, we can elect to use a rehab facility near our home for a while yet.

-If all goes as above, we'll discharge Thursday afternoon and stay at the hotel Thursday night. Then rest Friday and go to tae kwon do in Sugarland Friday night as a "test flight" for long-distance driving—it's a 45-minute drive one way. If that goes well, we'll head home Saturday morning.

-Fingers crossed...

04 May 2010 at 11:25am

Exactly one month ago today I was packing the car for our trip
here—our one-week trip that we'd done precisely the same way
twice before. What could POSSIBLY go wrong???

04 May 2010 at 11:39am

He CAN eat, and he WILL eat if food is placed in front of him. He
just doesn't have the wherewithal yet to initiate the steps to do for
himself, and his nature is to always answer, "No thanks, I'm fine"
when asked about anything.

So the staff shrugs and says, "He's fine. He said so." It's only his
mean wife who will say," Look, this is lunch. EAT IT".

It was also his wife who discovered something else. I placed a
menu in his hands and said, "Pick something out—what looks
good?"

He looked from me to the menu and back with irritation. Then he
thrust it back at me and turned away.

I asked if he wanted to read his book and handed it to him. He
opened it up and stared at it, concentrating mightily.

It was upside down.

My literate, brilliant husband, who owns and loves over 1,000
books, has forgotten how to read.

04 May 2010 at 2:26pm

Okie dokie. Ward's surgeon's PA just emailed me back. She said cardio doesn't really "assign" a doctor. They float through as needed and that the last notes from cardio entered into the computer were 4/26.

So who put him on Coumadin AND Lovenox???

A paraphrased transcript of the message I just left on the cardio clinic's voicemail-

"This is Sheri Dixon. My husband is Ward Dixon, Patient #******. He's inpatient right now in room P****. He was in ICU for heart failure post-op, and I haven't talked to a cardiologist in almost two weeks. The surgeon says the last cardio notes were on 4/26, but since then he's been put on Coumadin and the Lovenox has not been discontinued. I want a cardiologist to call me, with Ward's chart in front of him, TODAY before 5pm.
If I do not hear from a cardiologist TODAY, May 4th, I will be at the desk in the cardio department TOMORROW, and I have no problem at all with making a scene.

My phone number is ********** and I appreciate your help and look forward to talking to you. TODAY."

Too vague?

04 May 2010 at 9:32pm

So. At 4:45pm the nurse came into Ward's room and said, "Mrs. Dixon? The cardiologist is on the phone for you."

Damn. And I was so looking forward to visiting them in person tomorrow...

She was very nice and very apologetic and answered all my
questions:

-The Lovenox was to keep the graft from clotting.
-The Coumadin is for the re-formed clot that's already back and
what caused his a-fib after surgery. They want him on that for 6
months.
-They overlap because the Lovenox is short-acting and the
Coumadin takes a few days to kick in. What I witnessed was his
last Lovenox injection.
-They want to recheck him every two weeks to monitor the levels
and I said NO—he's got a very good cardio guy in Tyler who does
that and she said that's not in the notes.
-I said that's why I NEED their notes in hand and she agreed and
will deliver them tomorrow morning right to his room for me.

There. Was that so damn hard??? I thanked her for calling me, but
conveyed that I'd been requesting a call from them for TWO
WEEKS, and it was disappointing that it took me turning into a
frothing maniac to get a call.

Then the assisting surgeon came to the room and we discussed the
plan for discharge and after. They delivered a walker for him to
take with us, and there will be a wheelchair and shower chair/porta
potty delivered to the house before we get there. They will have
the home health care in place by tomorrow afternoon to start
Monday.

I talked to Ward about getting the brain scan—told him they
wanted it to have a "baseline" for his next checkup in July since
the only other one they have was before surgery and he said, "That
sounds like a good idea." He remembers what a CAT scan is, and I
told the doctor to schedule it for as early in the morning as possible
so he's as lucid as can be. I told him they'd be taking him out of the
room to do that and it was OK even though I wouldn't be there—
that it was going to be just a scan, like the many he's had before.

I think he'll be ok. He's not aggressive anymore; they'll just have to keep reminding him to hold still.

We did take Ward out for a Field Trip. He was antsy and wanted to GO SOMEWHERE, so we trundled him into a wheelchair and went to the hospital library where he found a book he's been wanting to read (that should help the next day and a half go quickly), then to the coffee shop for dessert and coffee, then

OUTSIDE to sit in the sunshine for the first time in a MONTH.

Less than 45 minutes. In a wheelchair. And he was totally pooped, got annoyed and said, "I need to lie down."

The furry monkeys remain his constant companions, and even though he was cheerful most of the day, twice Alec whispered to me, "He's not making a lick of sense." And he's right. He's still not.

Our trip home Saturday should be...interesting, but I hope totally uneventful.

05 May 2010 at 11:50pm

Talk to doctors at MDA in anticipation of discharge tomorrow? Check.
Talk to cardiologist in Tyler to make follow-up appointments for next week? Check.
Order medical alert/ID necklace for Ward to be delivered to the hotel Friday? Check.
Talk to social worker about home health care starting Monday? Check.
Go shopping for all food and gas we'll need till we bug outta Houston Saturday? Check.

Totally lose patience on the phone with husband who was pissed that we didn't see him today (we were there from 1pm-5pm) and that I didn't call him (I tried three times—he doesn't answer the phone) and said he didn't want to take a shower tomorrow (it's been a month since his last shower) and who's only response to, "Tomorrow you are getting discharged, which we've both been working for this last whole month" was to say, "Well, I don't know if I want to do that—I have to go make some coffee now..."?

Check.

It's gonna be a long few days.

06 May 2010 at 12:19am

Oh. And the CAT scan showed "nothing of note in his head." No change since the one before the first surgery. So no stroke—just "temporarily out of order."

06 May 2010 at 10:50am

Oh sure. NOW his memory comes back. He can't remember where he is yet or how to answer the phone, but he remembers me snapping at him last night and is pouting.

06 May 2010 at 10:34pm

Hey—guess who's right here next to me? In bed. At the hotel.

Ward. Ward Dixon.

What the hell am I doing on the computer?

Friday, May 7, 2010

Giving Credit Where Credit Is Due

When I was a child, my mother took me to Sunday School and church. Every single Sunday. I grew up in the church and believed what I was taught—even turning into a Sunday School teacher myself for a while.

I believed in the Bible. I believed that God was personal, and real, and cared about me and my family as individuals—like Santa Claus, he kept an eye on us all and took notes on our progress, our lives, our daily travails.

As I grew older, though, things didn't add up anymore. I had questions.

The questions were readily answered by Those Who Knew Better Than Me, and I believed the answers. Until I had a minute to think about them. Then they generally didn't make a damn bit of sense. Sometimes even less sense than the questions themselves.

Q: Why do newborn babies die? They haven't done anything wrong. Do they just get a minute on earth then an eternity in heaven?

A: It's all a part of God's Plan. Even so short, their lives touch those around them and teach those left behind important lessons.

Q: What about all those people who never get to hear about the story of Jesus? Do they still go to Hell even though it's not their fault they don't know?
A: Yes. Unfortunately they go to Hell. That's why it's so important that we send missionaries everywhere as soon as we can.

Q: Diseases like cancer—a lot of those people are good people who never did anything wrong—why should they suffer like they do?
A: No one is without sin. Life is full of opportunities to make ourselves right with the Lord.

Q: So, if Forgiveness and Redemption are given to anyone who truly regrets sinning and accepts Jesus as Savior, any old mass murderer can go to Heaven?
A: Yes. If a person truly accepts the Word, Heaven is theirs.

Q: If God can do anything, why does he let babies die, good people get cancer, and people kill other people in the first place?
A: Free Will—we must endure what comes and go to God of our own free will.

We watch *South Park*. Yes, it's a cartoon filled with profanity-spewing little children and Kenny always dies at the end of every show by some horrible means.

The writers also generally nail every social issue square on the head, from Gay Rights, to people with disabilities, to Saving the Rainforest, to the meltdown of our Financial Institutions, to any and all religions.

In one show, the parents of Stan are standing at his hospital bedside, comforting him while he endures the physical and emotional insult of having a bleeding hemorrhoid. He asks why a lot of very bad people seem to do OK, nay fabulously in life, while people like himself—a pretty good little boy—suffer.

They tell him the story of Job. Sort of a dare-fest between God and Satan. And Job loses. Loses his health, his home, and his family. But he never loses faith in God, who is pleased because He doesn't have to pay up to Satan. Stan rightly observes

"That's the worst story I've ever heard."

And decides then and there that there is no God.

I've just witnessed my husband endure trials that make what Job went through look like a day at the circus. For over a month, every time he started to get well, **BANG**—slapped back down by the Fickle Finger of Fate. Over and over and over again.

And much as I love our friends who love us and pray for us and who say, "God is so Good—to God goes the glory" every time Ward's made progress, I beg to differ.

I know, and am sorry, that they had nothing but prayers of encouragement when he got smacked down by one major surgery, then a week of medically-induced delirium, then another major surgery, then heart failure, then pneumonia—weeks of never-ending issues that were obviously NOT the Glory of God At Work. There were almost palpable pauses of disbelief on their parts as they grasped for something good to say, some comfort they could offer up to me from God as I watched my husband slip away violently time after time.

I believe there is a Higher Power. I believe there are consequences for how we act in this life and that how we live now will affect our next live(s).

But I believe that Ward is still here—very weak but still kickin'— partly because of the medical staff at the hospital, partly because his wife sat at his bedside and told him he was NOT allowed to die and he's as frightened of me as all the hospital staff learned to be, but mainly he's here because he has tremendous will, Herculean strength, and phenomenal courage.

Yes. God, or Mother Goddess (which I prefer), or the Higher Power may have gifted his soul with those attributes, but HE used them. HE, Ward, fought back with more endurance than anyone thought he had.

Mother Goddess gave his soul the gifts. He struggled damn hard to use them—to stay longer with me, and his son.

To Ward goes the glory—the admiration and the love.

He is more my hero now than he was before—something I told him the other day in the hospital while he was still fuzzy and trying to reconcile the loss of over a month of time from his consciousness and the loss of all his strength and muscle and about 30 pounds from his body, depressed and frustrated with them both—and our son looked at us and said, "Wow. That's saying A LOT."

Because he has always been, and is even moreso now, My Knight In Shining Armor.

07 May 2010 at 8:31pm

Day One of our Liberation.

Ward requested three things only:

1) To go to the bookstore, even for just a few minutes
2) COFFEE on-demand, all day long
3) Never being out of our sight or reach

Check, check, and check.

Using the walker to steady him, we also got him a lovely, if short shower. He's a New Man.

08 May 2010 at 9:08pm

HOME.

12 May 2010 at 12:41am

Well, we finally stood Ward on a scale. When he walked into MDAnderson on April 5th he weighed 185 pounds—and not a spare pound on him at 6'1."

Today, 41 days later, he weighs *148*. Gives him a better clue as to WHY HE'S SO DANG WEAK.

Physical therapy came by and did some very beginning work with him.

I told her that there was a very good reason my house looks like it does—we've been gone over a month—but god's truth is that it always looks this way so she shouldn't expect any better on subsequent visits...

Sunday, May 16, 2010

Just An Ordinary Day—How Extraordinary

We got back into town a week ago yesterday after over a month's forced interment in the Houston Medical District.

During that time, everything revolved around time spent at the hospital. Every minute, 24 hours a day seven days a week, was abnormal to our family. There were no daily farm chores, no big meals to be prepared—with just a kitchenette in the hotel room, there was no baking, roasting, broiling. The staff did the cleaning and linen laundry; our personal laundry was done in the hotel laundry room—no outside clothesline.

Most of our time was spent inside—the hospital, the hotel, the grocery store—and the times we made to spend outdoors were not fulfilling. There are no stars to be seen at night there, nor quiet to be had, even when surrounded by trees in a park.

The sounds, the smells, the oppressive closeness of millions of other people crammed into the cement jungle, weighed heavily on us. We yearned for our little town of 756 people, the countless stars at night, open windows, and the music of nature lulling us to sleep.

The first week we were home was devoted to catch-up and acquainting ourselves with some new, although temporary, realities.

"We'll have the home health people come give you a hand" seemed benign and helpful. What they don't tell you is that there is a nurse, a physical therapist, an occupational therapist, and a nutritionist—all with their own schedules that we must fit in between doctors' appointments and lab work.

I had a bi-monthly board meeting to prepare for and attend, and there were some pretty hefty changes at work that I had to institute, along with all the stuff that got way-sided while I was gone.

So this morning I got up at 7am and did what I most longed to do.

Not sleep in. Not put my feet up to read a book or watch a movie. Not go shopping or take a long bubble bath.

I did the morning chores, and delighted in the easy routine and the simple yet genuine pleasure of the animals at breakfast time.

I made a big brunch for my boys—pork chops, gravy, scrambled cheesy eggs, and biscuits, with lots of fresh ground coffee (cocoa for Alec), and delighted in the easy routine and the simple yet genuine pleasure of the boys at breakfast time.

I cleaned the guinea pigs and shuffled some around, separating out weanling babies and pregnant mommas, reflecting on almost 30 years of raising these endearing little critters.

I baked up a storm—two batches of triple fudge kickass brownies—one for us and one for a friend of ours who just had surgery on Wednesday, and an apple pie for the friend who ratted out which hospital the first friend would be at so I could surprise him and keep him company all day.

Cleaning the house is something that's not normally on my Favorite Things To Do list, but after being gone so long it's cathartic— possibly a form of "marking my territory"—to go through the house room by room, making sure to do those few things that really bother me when they're undone get done correctly, in a way only a Mom knows how to do.

For dinner, I made spaghetti sauce with Italian sausages and mushrooms, and homemade garlic bread—heavy on the Parmesan cheese.

All the cooking took just about every pot and mixing bowl I own, and it was good, the fact that we don't own a dishwasher not a burden, since washing by hand lets me remember where I got each mixing bowl, and appreciate the heavy smoothness of my grandmother's rolling pin.

And all day long I tended to the new puppy we got Friday, taking her outside where she demonstrated her obvious brilliance by pottying like a good doggie each and every time. While a new puppy might seem outwardly like the very LAST thing our family needs at this particular juncture, Fizzgig is a welcome diversion for Alec, for Ward, and for me- she's as sweet as she is smart, and has snuggled her way into our hearts in less than three days.

So I sat down here at 10pm—fifteen hours after rising this morning (the only times I've sat down otherwise all day were to pee)—and here I am.

I'm stiff, I'm exhausted, but after a week of being here, I finally feel like I'm home.

16 May 2010 at 9:06am

Ward's making astounding progress, which I tell him about a gazillion times a day. Although, since he can't REMEMBER the entire month+ that he was "down"—he remembers himself walking into the hospital at 185—he looks at himself now (he's still losing weight and is now 142) and says, "Sorry, this doesn't look like progress to ME."

We are using the wheelchair for any outings, since he gets dizzy easily and tires quickly, but at home he's walking around on his own.

His short-term memory problems are going away, and he's not nearly as fuzzy or confused as he was, Now we're sorting through what his brain says is "memory" and what may or may not be— just weird stuff mostly about places he's been, people we know, the stuff of dreams—but while the average dream takes only a few minutes for your brain to come up with while you're sleeping, his brain had an entire month pretty much unsupervised. Pretty. Bizarre. Stuff.

Oh. And it finally occurred to him yesterday to say, "I suppose everyone on the planet knows you were a meerkat, there were furry monkeys in my room, and that I saw a UFO with gun turrets." (Pause. Sigh) "Of COURSE they do."

The cardiologist said that, from the echo he did Friday, the heart failure appears to be more "event related" than chronic, and is already looking improved from the echo they did when he went into ICU—a very good thing. He's keeping Ward on the Coumadin for the clot and will repeat the echo the end of June.

He was very concerned (as am I) about the continued weight loss, and has Ward on two supplements a day in addition to three squares and as many snacks as I can get him to eat. His feeling is that Ward's body is in starvation mode and it's not absorbing most of what it's getting—explaining why his blood sugar is staying within range despite being on the Apple Pie Diet and getting NO insulin for the last three days. (When his night time reading was still only 135 after dessert and under 90 in the mornings, we stopped the insulin to avoid, yanno, diabetic coma.)

On account of we've had enough excitement for a while.

24 May 2010 at 11:50am

Good news—he's up to 145.

Bad news—his incision on his leg (where they harvested the graft) looks and feels infected.

There's no "opening" of the incision—it's still closed tight.

He's had a history of sealed abscesses.

The nurse today said it "might" be from the physical therapy making it inflamed.

We'll see.

02 June 2010 at 1:13am

One day left of the antibiotics they put him on-good old fashioned Amoxi—and though the infection doesn't look worse, it's not "all better" either, so we'll be sending another photo into the doctor.

Ward's working on his physical therapy every day and doing more every day. We're still working through the "memory or delusion" game.

And he's back down to 143, even after consuming a cream-cheese frosted carrot cake that made me gain five pounds just baking it.

He's so tired, so stiff, so painful, and not sleeping more than 20 minutes or so at a time.

We're both very discouraged and exhausted.

11 June 2010 at 1:07am

Yesterday was our 11th anniversary.

We go to the zoo (which was our first date 15 June 10ths ago) every year, but this year it was absolutely pouring buckets with thunder and lightning accompanying.

We'll go tomorrow, and I'll be pushing Ward in a wheelchair to do it, but by god we'll be at the zoo to commemorate our anniversary.

I'm so thankful that he's still with us, with me.

He's an amazing, strong, courageous and gentle man—my Knight in Shining Armor.

Always has been, always will be.

Friday, June 11, 2010

Today We Went to the Zoo

Sounds mundane, but in our case, it's not.

We went to the zoo for our first date—15 years ago yesterday.

Both newly divorced and pretty traumatized, we'd been friends— good friends, best friends—while we were each witnessing the deaths of our marriages, marriages that we both valiantly tried saving, even though we could see the terminal hopeless status of the other's situation. Afterwards, we fell apart in the aftermath and, though it looked a lot like "rebound," what we fell into was a deepening of our friendship, our very real concern for the other's happiness and well-being. We fell into love.

So we went to the zoo on June 10th, 1995, and about halfway through it Ward took my hand in his.

Even though we like the zoo, and go to the zoo several times a year, we always go to the zoo on June 10th.

We went to the zoo alone the first few years, but then had company—first a tiny baby of 4 months, and each year a bigger and bigger boy—this year a young man of 10 almost as tall as myself.

We went to the zoo in the rain at least once, speed walking through the deserted park with the animals peering out at us from their shelters, amused and bemused.

We went to the zoo when we were both employed and I'd pick up lunch, meet Ward at the picnic tables, inhale the food and barrel non-stop around the familiar route before a quick kiss and pointing our cars back to work.

Yesterday was June 10th. It was pouring rain. The rain gauge a few miles from here read 5.6 inches in less than 24 hours, though I've heard rumor of closer to 7 inches. There was thunder and lightning and we did not go to the zoo.

Today we went to the zoo.

Ward has endured so much these last few months. Less than eight weeks ago, medical personnel were encouraging me to put him in a nursing home, and a wheelchair has taken up residence in the trunk of our car. He's painfully thin and fragile looking, tires very easily, and is in almost continuous discomfort.

Today my husband walked around the zoo, refusing to use the wheelchair.

And I marvel in every tiny miracle and cherish my husband and my son—both so courageous and kind, intelligent and hilarious—

and though it seemed like the most normal average thing for a family to be there, walking around looking at the animals and enjoying sno-cones and animal crackers, it WAS a miracle to us, and not a tiny one, because there were more than several moments over the last few months when we were deep in the bowels of the cancer hospital that I couldn't hope, couldn't imagine, couldn't even aspire to think that we'd get another chance to say, casually

"Today we went to the zoo."

Monday, June 21, 2010

Beyond Father's Day

My older two children—the ones that aren't children anymore, being all grown up and whatnot—are products of my first marriage.

This "new" child—a mere 10 years old—is a product of my third marriage.

My husband (the third one—the GOOD one) has no other children, even though he had a former wife. When I expressed my desire (pun intended) to have another child before it was too late—I was looking the big Four O straight in the eyes—he said, "I don't know what the big deal is—any animal can reproduce".

About a year later he found out what the Big Deal is. Actually, the first time he felt that little critter kicking and punching inside me he started getting an inkling of the Big Deal-edness of the whole thing.

So we have this boy.

When a lot of men, especially those who've never had to share their wives with anyone else, have children, they are adamant about the baby sleeping IN THE CRIB.

We had a nursery set up in the big bedroom next to the kitchen. Three rooms away from our room.

Ward said, "You can't put that baby in there—he's spent nine months right next to you and he'll be all alone way back there. In the dark." So that baby moved into the bed with us, and there were many times I'd wake up to see them staring solemnly at each other.

Ward's never talked down to Alec- has always treated him as another human—not a baby, possession or toy, and never an annoyance.

He has the patience that the saints WISH they had.

So, wait.

YESTERDAY was Father's Day, what's the lame idea of writing about this NOW?

Today we went in for the initial consultation with the occupational therapist for Ward's outpatient treatments, and though he's still almost 50 pounds underweight with all the weakness, lack of stamina, and strength that go along with that, the main concern is his right shoulder.

Not this surgery (either one), but the LAST surgery over 2 years ago, they harvested a muscle from his back for the graft (the graft that failed necessitating THIS surgery/surgeries). This muscle holds the shoulder blade in place. When he had things like tissue and muscle back there, it was apparent that there were issues with that area. Truth told, he was supposed to go for physical therapy at the time, but he was still frantically trying to hold onto his job for the insurance he so clearly needed to have, so he/we blew it off.

Now, with nothing there but literally skin and bones, it's clear that he's really compromised in that shoulder—the blade pops out of place with little provocation and the entire area hurts like a son of a bitch most of the time.

So the therapist measured his reach, mobility, and strength, and recorded all of it. He had to fill out a ream of paperwork telling how difficult it is (on a scale of 1 to 5) to do things like lie down, kneel, balance, and go up and down stairs, etc. ad nauseum.

At the end of the session, she asked him, "Mr. Dixon—do you have any questions? Is there something in particular you want to be able to accomplish at the end of our working together?"

Ward loves to walk, to hike, to camp, to garden, to work on our property, to travel and sight-see everything from National parks to museums, and I expected him to answer with any of these things.

But he was quiet, head down for a moment, then he looked past me to Alec—obliviously reading his latest Star Wars novel—and he softly asked

"Do you think I'll be able to throw a ball again?"

Thursday, July 15, 2010

Kicking and Screaming—And Not in a Good Way

It's been so nice being home.

I've almost got the house back in order.

I've almost got work caught up.

Ward's healthier, heavier (up to 154 from his low of 141, but still 4 pounds shy of his hospital discharge weight of 158- a weight they classified as "extremely emaciated," and about 40 pounds shy of perfect), and he's getting stronger every day. The last few weeks, he has been going to out-patient physical therapy instead of having the home nurse come in.

Alec's getting back into the swing of school, art class, tae kwon do, and chores.

Yep, sure has been nice.

Time to go.

Nine hours from now, we'll be loading the car and heading back to Houston via Jackson, Mississippi (I know the abbreviation, I just like typing the whole word) where Alec will compete in the World ITA Championships—his 3rd world championship tournament and his 10th (I think) tournament in 4 years.

Then we'll head to Houston for re-checks and lab work and scans on Monday, Tuesday, and Wednesday.

So this week has been about collecting our house sitters, getting work situated to work without me for another week, all the mess that goes with leaving home for more than a day.

I've not had a chance to do a lot of news-scanning or thinking about much other than those tasks at hand—things to keep my son's life as normal as possible, my farm cared for and my employment justified, for Ward to once again endure things that we hope with all our hearts and minds will show and reassure us that my husband's cancer has not returned, that he is healing properly, that we'll be safe to come home till the next scans in four to six months.

As we've lived now for years—from scan to scan. Appointment to appointment.

Little things frighten me. Like the incision from this last surgery on Ward's neck that refuses to heal.

Because life is so fragile, no matter how big we try to make ourselves appear.

Typing this tonight, bone tired yet not ready for sleep, I listen with half an ear to some Celebrity News Show, and they've got close-ups of poor misunderstood Lindsay Lohan getting sentenced to 90 days in jail for being a terminal, perennial screw-up.

She's in tears and so frightened at the prospect of incarceration. For 90 days.

And I confess to being less than charitable.

I want to slap her upside her spoiled little head and tell her to stop sniveling and get her sorry little ass to jail. Then to rehab. Then, if she's very lucky and smartens up, on to the rest of her life.

90 days?

A walk in the damn park.

19 July 2010 at 9:53am

Alec and I are camped out on the 6th floor of the Mays Clinic—got our comfy chairs by the window and our computers plugged in and our feets up.

One benefit of having literally acres of unused waiting areas.

We got into Houston at midnight-fifteen and by the time I got the car unloaded and Fizzgig unwound it was 2am. Our wake-up time of 5:30 came up awfully quick behind that.

Ward had blood work at 7am and is in having a PET scan till about 10 or so. Then a CT scan at 11:30 and then he can EAT.

Then we'll head back to the hotel and I'll do some laundry and maybe catch a nap before dinner with a friend tonight and (if Alec's awake enough for it) training at the tae kwon do school in Sugarland.

Little Fizz has turned out to be a great traveler. Her basic temperament is so laid back, even as a puppy, she's happy wherever you say she's supposed to be. Getting her as a pup meant we could train her to sleep in her "hidey hole" (carrier), so traveling is easier than it was with Spooj—Spooj LOVED road trips, but hated being in a crate, so we'd have to leave her in the car (impossible here except for wintertime) or at a kennel—hotels frown on leaving dogs loose in the room while you're gone.

Fizzgig's only drawback is she's timid of new big things and loud noises, but she's getting better the more I expose her to that stuff. She's not but four months old, and so smart—one of those dogs you can just look in the eyes and TALK to; not teach commands to, but explain what and why and you can see them mulling it over in their heads and considering the merit of your request. Other than Spooj and the pyrs, I've never had dogs like that. It takes some getting used to...

Everything about her is soft. Even when you pick her up, she's not rigid like dogs normally are; she's slinky—like a cat, she kinda melts in your arms. But she's got that terrier solidness too. Hard to explain, but so soothing for Ward and so comforting for Alec.

And she's filling in, bit by bit, by the strength of her character and her irresistible muppet-ness, that huge gaping hole Spooj left when she died last fall- she stayed by my side for 15 years, her poor old body finally giving out to liver disease.

20 July 2010 at 9:01am

I do worry about Alec, and more than a little. He takes very seriously what he believes is his role to take care of US.

He worries and frets and has many fears about our health and the future—and although he KNOWS he can talk to us about anything, he hesitates to do anything to upset us or that he thinks we'll interpret as us failing him as child.

There's a counselor at MDA he really likes and whom he talks to about "stuff." She deals only with the children of cancer patients, and is a warm, funny, and fun woman. He spent about an hour with her yesterday, and we can see a difference in his demeanor—more relaxed, less anxious. Miss Martha is available to him via email all the time, and we try to get them together every time we're here for at least a little bit.

But mostly he has great compassion and empathy—traits that he comes by naturally, but that have been honed to a fine point because of our family circumstances.

Today's agenda—the pain doctor at 10:30 to see if there's anything else he can pull out of his hat for Ward's constant ache at the grafted area (which goes all the way to the top of his head, back to his ear, and even makes his teeth hurt on that side), and now the added muscle/joint pain from both his debilitating hospital stay and the physical therapy to reverse the weakness and emaciation. He can't take Tylenol, codeine, ibuprofen, aspirin, or morphine. Doesn't leave a whole lot...

Then to try to find the Thai restaurant Alec and I ate at after the dragon boat races. Name? No. I don't remember its name, why? Ummm. No. Not the corner it was on either. It's just a tiny hole in the wall place downtown in the 4th largest city in the US. How hard can that be to find???

Then to the Museum of Natural Science to see Lois, the Corpse Flower, who only blooms every few years.

And I think probably to the Chocolate Bar on Alabama St. for "dinner."

Sounds like a pretty full day.

20 July 2010 at 9:25pm

It's the Nit Noi Cafe on Main. We managed to find it by driving to where the dragon boat races were held and working our way out from there—we knew it was within a few blocks of the landing since we walked there.

The pain management doctor gave us a new plan. There's an extended-release form of the Tramadol that Ward's been taking— so something long-acting rather than to take as-needed for the sharp pains. If the long-acting doesn't completely take care of it, he may add ONE of the short-acting forms to zap it.

Then we found the cafe and had a wonderful lunch, then drove all the way back to Sugarland where Alec trained for tae kwon do last night to retrieve his sparring gear—we're so used to leaving it at our club in Tyler it never occurred to any of us as we left last night that we didn't have it—then to see LOIS, who's almost open. Our tickets are good through midnight, so if the LoisCam shows her opening tonight, we'll go back. I promised the boys that in any case, if she's open before we leave tomorrow after our 8am appointment, we'll go back to see (and smell) her.

Then to the Chocolate Bar for tuxedo cheesecake and now we're at the hotel, vegetating till we get hungry enough to eat lunch leftovers for dinner...

20 July 2010 at 10:04pm

The food at the Nit Noi is really, really outstanding—it's Alec's new favorite restaurant.

The bestest part—Ward across the table from me. Last time it was just Alec and me. Ward was fresh out of ICU and didn't know anything about where he was or who I was, and Alec sat across the table from me and made me PROMISE that we'd bring daddy back here to eat.

And we did.

And it was an amazing moment to count blessings.

27 July 2010 at 10:52pm

…And in OTHER news—we got the call this afternoon, the one we look forward to every 4 months: "Mr. Dixon, there is nothing of note in your head."

Cancer-wise, we're good to go till November.

Thursday, July 29, 2010

And Just Like That…

…Three good things in a row.

Three REALLY good things in a row.

Our banker gave us the thumbs-up to go ahead and build our little cabin on our land—something that's been on hold pending the sale of our current house that's been for sale for FIVE YEARS, right after we bought our "we could live here forever" land three miles from where we are now. And while it would be better to have our current house sold before building, our debt to income ratio INCLUDING both house payments (old house plus new yet-to-be-built house) was only off by 3 (three) points. That three points, coupled with the 2 (two) points our credit score was lacking, were all that's been holding this project up, and bless his heart, our banker shook my hand and told me that they'll do it in-house because we've been good customers for over 15 years and it's just time for us to do this.

And the benefit is that we get to build the new place, move stuff over there that we KNOW we want to keep, sort through the rest here at the old place, have a big honkin' yard sale, and donate/dumpster the rest without any "live in an apartment/store all our stuff" phase that new-home construction after a house sale generally entails. Which is good, because I truly don't think either Ward or I could survive that mess.

We may have buyers for our current house, and they are not in a hurry to move out of their old house, which would allow us to do exactly the above scenario, then transition smoothly (two words that are rarely found next to each other in our family conversations for most of the last decade) into selling this house.

On our way to dinner with the above folks, the doctor at MDAnderson called to give us the results of Ward's recent scans— All Clear. No cancer there, they'll see us in four months for the next scans.

That.

That right there was the Other Shoe I was mortally afraid would be not just dropped, but also slammed up against our heads, in the wake of the Loan Approval/Pending Buyers One-Two that we'd received earlier.

And it didn't happen.

The Good kept coming.

We met our neighbors at the restaurant and I told them the Three Good Things. They grinned from ear to ear and asked me, "Can you stand so much good news all at once?"

I told them that quite frankly it scared the shit outta me.

Dot looked at me and said, "Just GO with it."

And I'm trying. I'm taking deep breath after deep breath and each one clears a few more moldy cobwebs from my lungs, from my heart.

Maybe it's finally Over. Maybe that almost six weeks in Houston filled with fear and terror and sheer relentless hell were the Final Tidal Wave of the eight years that started with, "It's just a little skin cancer," and my family has finally landed, tattered, worn, twitchy, but still firmly intact, into the Calmer Safe Harbor of the Sea of Life.

Ward poked Alec and said, "Look at your mom, son."

Alec, a little startled, whispered, "What's wrong with her?"

Ward said, "Nothing son—she's smiling."

And I am.

Tuesday, August 17, 2010

Getting Away With Murder

I know the worst of that whole Abysmal April was the time period after hearing the words, "When we tried to wake him up from anesthesia he went into heart failure and stopped breathing." Most specifically, the 12 hours or so after that, when they really didn't know if he'd ever wake up again. If they'd ever be able to turn off the machines breathing and beating for him without marking the time and covering him in a sheet.

People say something horrible is "like a nightmare," but when you're really truly wide-awake living it, you pray for a nightmare to give your life a little levity.

And during that time, four thoughts ran through my head over and over and over again without stopping, on a mental loop trying to lasso my sanity.

One: what will I tell Alec? Ward's his Hero. How can I raise him all by myself?

Two: Ward told me before this surgery that he'd be OK. He said, "It'll be alright. I'm going to be fine. You and I have a lot we have to do yet." Ward has never lied to me in over 15 years, and I was by god going to hold him to this one.

Three: Please. As in a prayer. One word asking that I not have to...ever...not now, not ever... go to the computer, log in and type

"I am a widow."

Four: Visuals of our friends Sunni and Jim, Sharlotte and Edward. Quiet, kind, patient Jim. Ornery, exasperating, kind Edward. Sunni and Sharlotte alone now—just in the past few months having typed "I am a widow" into the blank of their lives that asks "marital status."

It was this last thought that was the most terrifying. There was basically nothing wrong with either Jim or Edward and they had nothing in common health-wise with Ward—Jim was younger and Edward older—except for one thing. They both (like Ward) went into the hospital with something fixable. But Jim and Edward never made it out again.

Jim went into the hospital following a mild stroke. He ended up contracting pneumonia and dying there.

Edward went into the hospital with intestinal problems that required some surgery. He ended up aspirating during a post-op MRI, contracted pneumonia and died.

Ward was much more fragile. Much less healthy BEFORE his "alarming event."

He'd entered the hospital after numerous infections and bleeding episodes, but was deemed well enough for the surgery to repair the failed graft that was the source of the infections and bleediness.

He went from a long complicated surgery
To a very bad drug reaction
To an emergency surgery
To his heart and lungs saying, "That's it—we're out"
To mechanical support in ICU
To pneumonia
To staph infections
And then, amazingly

To a slow, torturous, frustrating, frightening, but hallelujah-praise-whoever's-up-there recovery.

Ward was lucky. Ward IS lucky. Alec and I are lucky.

And it so easily could've slipped quietly, quickly, and fatally in the other direction. As it did for our friends. Not people in the news. Not abstract figures or names in the death notices. To our friends.

That's a few months behind us, and Ward's still making slow but sure recovery, so what in blue blazes am I doing re-hashing all this mess???

We've got a guinea pig show coming up, and Sunni and Jim are guinea pig friends. We've stayed more than once at their home and cherished every minute we've ever had with them.

I talked to Sharlotte today—she lives just up the road from us and we buy hay from them. She and Edward have always been there for us for any reason and at any time.

So I had both couples on my mind lately. Couples that aren't anymore. Not because of natural causes or an accident or because they didn't make it to the hospital in time.

They died BECAUSE they were at the hospital. And not tiny little bohunk boonies hospitals—Sunni and Jim live in Austin and Edward went to our large regional hospital (clever hint given two paragraphs down). Just as Ward almost died directly BECAUSE of what was done or not done for him or to him at MDAnderson Cancer Center, one of the premier hospitals in the world.

And it's not just some freak bad karma following my friends and me around, zapping our men folk—this shit happens every day, in every hospital in this country.

Way back when we were just starting on our Cancer Family Adventure, I was waiting for Ward to get his hydrotherapy at our large regional hospital. Let's call it Trinity Mother Frances in Tyler, Texas. To pass the time, I went to the cafeteria for a cuppa coffee.

On every table were little placards- colorful cardboard centerpieces to both inform and make dining more enjoyable. That was a very long time ago, but the gist of the placards was this:

Hospital Death Awareness Week [fill in the dates]
A week of educational seminars focusing on lessening the
occurrence of death due to hospital-contracted conditions
[Listing of educational seminars]
Trinity Mother Frances Hospital 20XX goal: LESS THAN 1,500.

I re-read it a few times, in different light and at different angles
because there was no way I could fathom

a) That this was something they'd put in the PUBLIC cafeteria for
loved ones of patients to peruse and
b) That "Less than 1,500" was something to shoot for, death-wise.

And I guess, from the safety of this far away from our own near-
death experience, I can breathe, close my eyes, and get truly and
totally pissed off about a hospital that thinks "less than 1,500" is
not only acceptable, but admirable.

That healthy people can go into a hospital in good faith and with
no real concerns and not come out.

And that the hospitals are not accountable.

They may express concern. The individual players may grieve
right with you, because I really believe that most of them ARE
there to heal, to care for, to nurture other humans, and the problem
is that the environment they have to do it in is toxic and/or
managed not by health professionals but by accountants and
insurance companies and/or the systems used to keep records is
ridiculously cumbersome and archaic.

But when you enter a hospital in America for any reason
whatsoever, you must sign a little paper before a doctor will even
come into the same room with you. That paper says that you give
the hospital and its staff permission to treat you as they see fit.
That the outcome of your visit may or may not be favorable to you,
and may end in disfigurement, a worsening of your condition, the
addition of new conditions or possibly death.

It's a permission slip.

It's a golden ticket.

For getting away with murder.

And I think of Jim and Edward and Sunni and Sharlotte. I look at Ward—the shadow of what he's been through hangs on him, dragging him down, and he fights his way through it every single day for the last 3 months and for many months to come.

And people who've never skated that close to the edge shrug apologetically and say, "Well, what can you do?"

And people who've tipped into that frigid bottomless pit go to the phone book and call a lawyer and see what they can do. And the answer is, "Not much."

We actually saw a lawyer way back when we found out that Ward's surgeon here in Tyler was well aware that she did not get all the cancer when she enucleated his eye, even though she told us she did, and even though they radiated the snot out of the area (they told us) "just in case."

Although the lawyer was sympathetic, and he AND his medical advisor said she'd not done the right thing, he declined the case. He said the only cases he could afford to take were what he called "jaw-droppers"—something that a jury would just freakin' not believe—and that had ended in death.

And we told him that while money would sure be nice to pay off all the subsequent "this was caused by her actions/inactions" expenses that had already totaled into the tens of thousands of dollars, our main goal was to make her stop.

Make her stop and THINK before saying, "Oh yes—I do these all the time."

And I believe that's all most people who bring lawsuits for medical negligence want—because no money on earth will fill the hole losing your spouse, your parent, or your child leaves in your heart.

Just STOP and think before doing something, or before blowing something off.

Because you've got someone's life in your hands.

And even though we've signed the permission slip, you need to do everything in your power to not have to use it.

Monday, September 20, 2010

Houston Haiku Trilogy

My knight in shining armor
Sleeps just to my left.
Watching him breathe calms my heart.

My brave son and his Fizzgig
Sleep just to my right.
Stork legs, short legs, feet and paws.

I'm exhausted past slumber
Yet sleep just won't come
For Wife, Mom, and Worrier.

Please keep my family in your thoughts and yes, even prayers, as we once again enter the maws of MD Anderson...again. Tomorrow and Wednesday are "routine" appointments, but for some reason we're a little twitchy just being here.

Friday, September 24, 2010

Internet Medical Research + Midnight:Thirty = Nothing Good Ever

So there's this spot.

It's on Ward's neck, right about where they harvested a vein for this latest graft. Actually, that's not entirely true.

That spot (hereafter referred to as "the area") has just sort of been there all along after surgery—I'm not really sure, though, since his entire body was so ravaged away back in April that the area was most likely the BEST looking place on his entire body for a good while.

About the size of a dime, give or take since it scabs and opens, scabs and opens, it's never really gotten infected, but never really healed over.

The doctors looked at it in July and said, "Well, looks like post-surgical trauma. It should heal—we'll keep an eye on it." They mainly want to keep an eye on it since it's right over what's left of the same muscle that grew his cancer.

But at the time, they scanned it and said, "No cancer."

Complicating matters is that that side of Ward's head has had its nerve endings (and everything else) all messed up and rearranged, and the area is where he naturally rests his head in his hand. So the area is apparently just irritating enough for him to bother it, but doesn't have enough feeling for him to tell just how much damage he's doing to it.

I've bugged him. Alec's bugged him. Every time we see his hand wander up there, we throw something at him. I've stopped just short of getting a spray bottle.

The obvious answer, cover the area, I've been loathe to do since that skin is SO delicate—any adhesive used to keep bandaging on there would've most likely torn off more skin when removed. And that's not the direction we want to go.

So we've gone back and forth, and it got better and worse, and we were told it would most likely heal—that we needed to remember that Ward's not only diabetic but also on Coumadin—both things that make healing a slow going proposition.

But here's the thing.

Everywhere else on Ward is healed beautifully from that month-plus long assault on his person. The graft is perfect, the incisions are solid, the donor sites are almost invisible, and even when Fizzgig scratches him in her puppy exuberance and he walks around with a paper towel dripping blood for an hour, those spots are 150% All Better No More Boo Boo within a week.

And then the second spot appeared a few weeks before these appointments.

Just to the face-side of the area and looking like it's Evil Looking-Glass Twin.

Which is the main reason I was sleepless in Houston and writing Haiku earlier this week.

The cancer doctor said, "Well, the scans from July show 'something'—probably scar tissue, but definitely not normal tissue. We can do two things—we can make sure you keep that covered to rule out self-mutilation, and if it's not completely healed in three weeks, you come back for a consultation and biopsy with the dermatologist OR we can just do the biopsy now."

I was ready—just show me the needle, hand me a syringe, and I'll get it myself ya'll just hold that man down for a sec.

Ward said, "Not so fast, Over-reaction Mama."

Being as he's the patient, and my beloved husband, and just an all-around better and more sensible person than I am, we're going with the Option of Least Invasiveness for now, which the doctor never would've even offered if he thought for a second that three weeks would make any difference. I know that because that's exactly what he told us in a quiet calming voice as they were gently tightening the ties on my strait jacket...
As we were leaving, we were offhandedly asked the last time Ward's seen a dermatologist. As in, "You ARE seeing a dermatologist on a regular basis for an all-over check for more skin cancer, right?"

Ummm...no. We're not. We were never told to. We come to MDAnderson every 4-6 months for THEM to keep on top of it and FOR GOD'S SAKE NO ONE HERE EVER TOLD US WE NEEDED TO DO THAT!!!

(Those strait jackets at MDA are really top notch—never even loosened an inch...)

The bandaging they prescribed is something called Tagaderm—sort of sticky cellophane, cut to fit and applied over the area. They said, "Well, try this—but it doesn't breathe so if the area gets oozy or yacky or otherwise more disgusting than it already is, be sure to take it off". But no other options. Thanks.

Within eight hours, the area was oozy and yacky and more disgusting than it already was, so we removed the Tagaderm, thankful that we hadn't already spent $15 on four little pieces of it at the drugstore.

So...what to do what to do what to do about keeping the area covered yet breathing?

I've got almost 30 years working in the veterinary field, so I fell back on what came naturally to me and slapped a cervical collar on him.

What the Sam Hell does any of that have to do with the title of today's post, you crazy old broad???

Just this.

Last night I surfed the interwebs while my family slept (except for the Mutant Cat from Hades—it never sleeps) and came across some interesting yet horrifying things:

-The area does, in fact, look suspiciously basal cell-ish
-A reminder that while basal cell doesn't usually metastasize, it can be "aggressive and problematic at point of origin"

and my favorite

-Of patients who are treated for basal cell, over 50% will have it recur near the original site within five years.

Today the area looks some better. I'm letting Ward not wear the collar unless we start to see him pecking at it again and/or during the times he would normally be resting his head in his hand—watching TV, surfing the 'net, or in the car.

All I can say is, those sum-bitches better keep on healin', because my family has got a house to build, things to do, places to go, people to see, and none of it includes any more incarcerations at the cancer hospital.

Tuesday, October 12, 2010

Lists

My world, like most people's, is filled with lists.

Grocery lists, shopping lists, errand lists, chore lists.

Lists on the telephone, the computer, typed neatly and posted on the wall, or scratched onto the back of a junk mail envelope using a pen that's out of ink.

There's a running list on the Notepad feature of my phone—stuff we need at the store...next time we're there.

I travel at all times with two bags plus my purse—my workbag and the "house building stuff" bag.

The workbag is a misnomer since it's got the stuff (and lists) for the taekwondo club Alec belongs to in one section—I'm the treasurer of the club. It's got our bills to be paid and calls to be made (in list form) in another section. And there is work stuff in there, too—schedules, calls, orders, lists.

The house bag has all the details of our building project— contracts, blueprints, receipts, business cards, and phone numbers. And many. Many. Lists.

On one of my lists is the directive to "clean out all drawers and surfaces." This is daunting because we're packrats, every one of us. But I need to clean those areas in order to get to the furniture we want to move, and this whole Moving Thing is an exercise in cleaning out the old, shaking off the cobwebs from our previous life, starting anew and all that drivel.

Here's the thing.

I'm finding, tucked into drawers and cupboards and files...a lot of old lists.

And that slows me down, because they must be read, remembered, and validated before either being tossed out or saved.

I'm not talking about old grocery lists; those are easy to discard. I'm talking about the many, many lists and plans and letters and drawings that led up to the reality of the house we're now building (these get saved).

I'm talking about Christmas wish lists, painstakingly written out in ever-more-legible handwriting by our son.

I wonder, now that he "knows about Santa" will there be a wish list this year?

I remember the conversation that led up to the very large next step of being grown-up:

"Mom—is Santa real?"

"Well, son, what do you think?"

"I don't know- that's why I'm asking you."

"Son, Santa is the spirit of giving. In that respect he's very real, and always will be."

"Soooo...he's you."

"Yes, dear."

"But mom?"

"Yes, dear?"

"I always put the really expensive stuff on Santa's list because I knew you couldn't afford it."

"Yes dear."

"Mom? I always got those expensive presents."

"I know dear."

Pause

"So you're Santa."

"Fraid so."

"All this time you've been Santa."

"Yep."

Pause

"Mom?"

"Yes dear?"

(Whispered) "Does dad know?"

(Whispered) "No dear. Let's not tell him—he's had a rough couple of years..."

The Christmas lists ALWAYS get saved.

There are worn, stained mapquested route pages from every epic journey we've taken ("Family Vacation" just doesn't cover the scope of how we travel...). Those get saved.

So I was actually enjoying my little jaunt down List Memory Lane.

Until.

Going through a pile of stuff we brought back from the last trip to MDAnderson, I found The List.

It's dated April 29, 2010, about a week before Ward's discharge. It's from the Social Worker at MDA. See, he'd reached a point where he didn't NEED to be in the hospital anymore, but physically he couldn't walk more than a few steps and mentally he was still really, really fuzzy. Really. He was weak and fuzzy from drug reactions and weeks of intensive care and two major surgeries and heart failure and pneumonia and he was just plain wore out.

They told me that they were stumped that he was not improving from the point he was at, and they hinted and inferred that where he was might be all the better he got— wheelchair bound and mid-Alzheimer's.

There was concern that I wouldn't be able to take care of my husband, wouldn't be able to handle his handicaps in our home. It was strongly suggested that he not come home, at least for a few weeks. Or months. Or however long it took for him to be more "mentally reliable" and for him to get stronger.

And they handed me The List.

"Nursing Homes and Rehabilitation Facilities in the Greater Houston Area."

But I couldn't, wouldn't do it.

I just couldn't merge together the repeated assurances that, the more he was surrounded by familiar people, the quicker he'd recover, with the idea of putting him in a COMPLETELY new environment, filled with all new people he'd never seen before.

He's my husband. No one knows him, loves him, and cares about him more than I do, and I was determined to bring him home.

Because I work flexible hours, and because Joe was here to assist physically if needed and to be watchful when I had to be at work—

meaning Ward was never alone at home— we were approved to come home. All of us. Together.

Five months later, Ward's pretty much back to his brilliant, funny, beloved old self. His weight is coming up nicely from the over-40-pounds underweight he left the hospital carrying, and thanks to physical therapy he's gaining strength steadily.

I looked at The List, transfixed, paralyzed, instantly awash with the emotions the first reading of that self-same list filled me with— sadness, worry, fear.

Bleakness.

I showed The List to Ward. So much of that time was filled with stuff he can't remember, stuff he remembers but never happened, strangeness. I showed it to him so he'd know I wasn't exaggerating when I told him it was recommended that I put him in a nursing home.

Then I firmly and deliberately folded The List in half, and tucked it into The Trash.

12 October 2010 at 1:30am

Our appointments went mostly OK.

The graft is perfect.

Mentally he's 99% and physically, with the help of twice-weekly physical therapy, he's about 65% of where he was before surgery in April—a huge gain from the 10% (or less) on both he came out of the hospital with.

He's gained over 25 pounds back—over halfway to normal.

The biggest concern is the spot(s) on his neck—the one(s) on the same muscle his cancer was on. We didn't really notice it (them) till July. I guess he was so beat up in April/May that a little spot (the size of a dime) looked pretty good.

But. It's not on a suture line. If it were, that could be explained away as surgical insult/irritation. One issue is that the tissue on that whole side of his head has been so torn up and pieced back together that it's just irritating enough to bug him, but the nerve endings are numb enough that he doesn't realize how much damage he may be doing himself there.

Alec and I both get after him, stopping just short of spritzing him with a spray bottle (like keeping a cat off the countertops). I'm loathe to put any adhesive over it since the skin is so fragile there.

I actually went to the pharmacy and got the widest whiplash collar I could find.

Hey, I've worked for veterinarians for over 25 years—it's what I know...

What worries me (and the doctors) is that one spot will heal, and another will come up right next to it, and then repeat. He's been down to one spot, but has had as many as three.

The doctor said, "Well, you can make a conscious effort to NOT BUG THEM and see if they do heal for good. If they don't heal in, say, three weeks, you MUST come back for a biopsy."

Me being me, I wanted to do the biopsy right then, but Ward insisted we wait.

And I asked the doctor if it would make a difference. He said it wouldn't, or he'd never have given us the option. If it IS a recurrence, it "should" be the same kind of cancer, which rarely metastasizes but can be "problematic and aggressive at point of origin" (YA THINK???) and should be "fairly easy and straightforward" to take care of.

Everything in me wanted to know NOW what we're dealing with, but Ward almost never butts heads with me, and I have to respect his wishes. I know what he's thinking—he later told me his reasoning. Our house project has been delayed over and over again due to cancer and the aftereffects and he refuses to have it stopped literally mid-build.

So I bullhead through every single day and get after the various people involved and they all know that we're dealing with way more than merely a "wanna get our house finished" deadline.

It's why we went from closing to ready for the shell in 12 days.

Ward's 3 weeks are up tomorrow and the spots are still there.

He keeps saying, "No—they're healing," but one will heal and another comes up. He refuses to go back to MDAnderson until the house is up.

I've started cleaning out the "stuff" of our lives that's accumulated for the last 15 years in this house and tonight I found the list the social worker at MDAnderson gave me just a week before he was discharged in May—the list of nursing homes in the Houston area they recommended I put him in since he was still so fuzzy and weak.

I just stood there with that in my hands and started shaking- I can't—WE can't—go through another bit like this past April...

So tomorrow I meet with the fence contractor and the well tester, and the barn goes up Friday. Everything to finish the inside once the shell is up is in our contractor's barn, and we're next in line once a log crew is free.

Alec's planning his Halloween party at the new place--hopefully the shell will be complete by then. If not, it'll be a slab party.

Every day my ear's on the telephone, my feet are on our property, and my eyes are on Ward's neck.

One day at a time.

12 October 2010 at 1:15pm

The hardest thing for me to do is to back off.

But yanno, Ward's had precious little control of anything the last few years, and specifically the last 6 months—he feels he CAN control getting his family under the new roof, safely, finally and at last.

If it's nothing- no harm no foul.
If it's something- they'll take care of it in a month or so.
If it's something bad- he's taken care of US.

Dr. Hanna is the head of the Head and Neck Department at MDAnderson. He's the one who found what everyone here at the regional hospital missed and we trust his opinion.

He said the scans show abnormal tissue in that area, but that there's been so much insult there it's not GOING to look normal. He said it doesn't scream CANCER to him, but if it doesn't heal, it needs to be checked.

I just came back from the property a little bit ago. The fence guys are staking out the goat paddocks. While they did that I hiked to the top of the hill—there's a grove of pines that's come up at the base of the big sweet gum tree and there's a clearing in there that's invisible till you're actually in it.

The grass has been mowed neatly by the deer.

The rain yesterday caused some sort of gnat hatch.
And there were hundreds of dragonflies dancing in the air,
catching lunch on the wing.

Deep breaths. Over and Over Again.

Wednesday, December 8, 2010

Confessions of the Lesser Parent

My husband is a wonderful father.

Right from the get-go, the second I went into labor and calmly
informed him, "You are to take my hand and not let go...till it's
over," and the man seriously did not so much as pee till 12 hours
later when Alec made his entrance into the world.

Oh, there was that one time that he dropped the baby on his head,
but not very far, and it WAS onto the carpeted floor.

But other than that, Ward's clearly the better parent.

Take a few nights ago.

Alec is sick—sore throat, fever, and headache—and it broke night
before last. Poor boy woke up twice in tears, which I know because
Ward joggled me and asked, "Is that Alec?"

The first time I surfaced to consciousness long enough to listen to
the low, mournful, repetitive noise coming from the direction of
my son's room, I said, "No- I think that's coyotes." before sinking
back into slumber. Some time later (not much later, maybe a few
minutes) I came fully awake since my nice warm husband wasn't
next to me anymore.

I stumbled into the next room where he was already ministering to our son—feeling his head, calming him down, and telling him it was going to be OK.

And while part of me searched for something that *I*, as The Mother, should be doing, the other part thought, "Cool. It's all under control and I can go back to bed now—my side of the bed is probably still warm".

See?

And that's just one example. I got a million of 'em.

Seriously.

2011

Thursday, January 20, 2011

Lucky Ducks

So, last week we were given the good news we hold onto every four months.

The cancer doctor said, "Mr. Dixon- there is nothing of note in your head," meaning, of course, that the cancer has not returned, and we are dismissed for another few months. The cancer doctor thinks the "nothing of note in your head" comment is wildly hilarious, as do we, so it's all good.

As an added bonus, he said we may stay away for six months now, since the cancer has been gone for almost four years. We are breathing a little easier, sleeping a little better, daring to feel a little more fortunate than we did before.

Luck is a funny thing.

Because shit just happens. It's easier, neater, more comforting to imagine and believe that Everything Happens for a Reason, but I'm thinking that most of the time it doesn't. Most of the time Shit Really Does Just Happen.

Good people get slammed with a lot of crap.

Bad people win the lottery.

There's no ulterior cosmic motive to it—no behind-the-scenes god knows all souls and rewards/punishes accordingly. This is Life. It's messy, beautiful, tragic, hilarious and almost completely random. And it's OK.When we were seeing the pain doctor last week, he asked for Ward's medical record number—at MD Anderson, you can forget your name, address, birth date, and social security number. You are known by your medical record number, and better have that baby memorized.

Ward's is very easy—a combination of only two numbers in a nicely arranged pattern.
So for almost four years, clerical and medical staff have all said the same thing:

"Wow. That's an easy number—how lucky for YOU."

And for almost four years, I've replied the same way:

"Yes. How lucky we are to have an easy-to-remember number at the CANCER HOSPITAL."

The reaction is generally nervous, self-conscious laughter on the part of the staff. The pain doctor, however, looked at me, then at Ward, and said, "Wow. She goes straight for the jugular, doesn't she?"

Ward smiled and said, "Yep. She's a mean 'un."

Pain doctor—"And I think she hit the carotid too..."

I just smiled sweetly and said, "Well, as long as I was already there- I like to be efficient".

And we all laughed.

Tuesday, January 25, 2011

"There May Be a Small Disruption of Service"

We're moved.

They came and took all our big heavy furniture and set it up in the new house—in and around the electrician still hanging fixtures and the contractors still putting up walls. It looks terrific—just like the house was custom designed for the furniture and people who live here. Which, of course, it was.

And after all the work, planning, hoping, blood, sweat, tears, delays, frustrations, and heartbreak, the new house is not everything I'd hoped it would be.

It's a thousand times more.

The friends and family who've been out to the new place have said it looks like us... and that they've never seen anything like it (does that mean we're weird?).

People HAVE to touch the logs—the logs with the bark still on them. There is something compelling, powerful, and comforting about the honesty of their non-conformist widths, shapes, colors, and flaws, and people feel the need to absorb some of that through their fingertips.

The naturally knotted and variegated wood on the ceilings and walls provide a never-ending exercise in visual interest. The rock fireplace (even though still a work in progress), with its free-form shape, begs to be patted like a huge, sturdy, protective dragon. Even the cement floor has shaded swirls and patterns—and all we did was seal it.

We all three of us wander around almost gingerly, as if, at any moment, it could disappear like Cinderella's pumpkin carriage.

But every morning we wake up and our house is still around us. Our family is still together and our house is still around us.

And we'll never, ever take either one of those seemingly simple occurrences for granted.

When we returned from our most recent appointments in Houston, we walked into the house and I immediately fell into Ward's arms in tears.

The entire way to Houston, I was terrified that they would tell us the cancer was back—because having this house at last was such a miracle.

The entire way home from Houston, I was terrified that the house would be gone when we got here—tornado, fire, something— because having him cancer-free was such a miracle.

"It's still here- You're still here"...and I couldn't stop shaking and crying.

07 May 2011 at 11:56pm

One year ago today, our family limped home from the hospital— weak, tattered, frazzled, and generally wore out.

We're better now.

What I DO know is that, while re-reading, and therefore mentally re-living, this stuff brings back a ton of really unpleasant feelers- fear, frustration, panic, anger, exhaustion—it's also so very real and important that I acknowledge that we're looking back at it from a place we only dreamed of a year ago. One where we are physically and mentally well, and—just the pure capital M miracle—that we ARE still a family, we ARE still together,

The nightmare did end.

Tonight I breathe deeply of the honeysuckle trailing the length and breadth of our 12-acre speck of heaven, filling lungs that have almost forgotten the smog and exhaust fumes and pre-breathed air already exhaled from the lungs of 4 million other people.

Almost.

Friday June 10, 2011

I Take You, Ward...

...To have and to hold, for better for worse, for richer for poorer, in sickness and in health, to love and to cherish, till death us do part.

We've run the Vow Gauntlet and come out the other side still strong, still together, and still very much in love.

You are, and always have been, my strength, my safety, and the calming force that keeps my head from exploding on a daily basis.

My knight in shining armor.

I did.

I do.

I always will.

For always and forever.

Happy Anniversary, Gomez.

AND THEY LIVED HAPPILY EVER AFTER.

Sheri Dixon lives with, loves, and cares for her family in the heart of the East Texas Pineywoods.

An Ol' Treehuggin' Hippiechick, all she's ever wanted to do when she grows up is to write.

Thanks to the encouragement and support of her family, prodded into action by passing the Big 5-0 recently, she's decided to concentrate on writing.

...But she steadfastly refuses to grow up.

CancerDance—a love story is her first book.

Please visit her at www.sheri-dixon.com